GLUTEN FREE COOKBOOK

A Sweet and Savory Guide You Must Have

(Easy, Healthy and Delicious Meals You'll Both Love)

Julie Cortez

Published by Sharon Lohan

© **Julie Cortez**

All Rights Reserved

Gluten Free Cookbook: A Sweet and Savory Guide You Must Have (Easy, Healthy and Delicious Meals You'll Both Love)

ISBN 978-1-990334-15-3

All rights reserved. No part of this guide may be reproduced in any form without permission in writing from the publisher except in the case of brief quotations embodied in critical articles or reviews.

Legal & Disclaimer

The information contained in this book is not designed to replace or take the place of any form of medicine or professional medical advice. The information in this book has been provided for educational and entertainment purposes only.

The information contained in this book has been compiled from sources deemed reliable, and it is accurate to the best of the Author's knowledge; however, the Author cannot guarantee its accuracy and validity and cannot be held liable for any errors or omissions. Changes are periodically made to this book. You must consult your doctor or get professional medical advice before using any of the suggested remedies, techniques, or information in this book.

Table of contents

Part 1 1
Introduction 2
Recipes 3
Grilled Marinated Shrimp 3
II. Barbecued Beef 4
III. Baked Kale Chips 5
IV. Roasted Yam and Kale Salad 6
V. Black Beans and Quinoa 7
VI. Caramel Pork Chops 9
VII. Roasted Brussels Sprouts 10
VIII. Roasted Garlic Cauliflower 11
IX. Roasted Cauliflower Soup 12
X. Buckwheat Crepes 14
XI. Honey-Roasted Cinnamon Walnut Butter 14
XII. Weight Watchers Cabbage Soup 16
XIII. Homemade Salsa 17
XIV. Roasted Broccoli with Lemon Garlic and Toasted Pine Nuts 18
XV. Crustless Spinach Quiche 19
XVI. Oven-Dried Tomatoes 20
XVII. Grilled Moroccan Chicken 21

XVIII. Cream of Broccoli Soup 22

XIX. Shrimp Scampi 24

XX. Watermelon Lemonade 25

XXI. Gluten-Free Pizza Crust 26

XXII. Marinated Olives 28

XXIII. Sweet Potato and Pumpkin Mash 29

XXIV. Jazzed-up Hummus 30

XXV. Coconut Brown Rice 31

XXVI. Roasted Pumpkin Seed Spread 32

XXVII. Zucchini Casserole 33

XXVIII. Black Bean Brownies 35

XXIX. Flourless Peanut Butter Cookies 36

XXX. Stuffed Peppers 37

XXXI. Rice Noodles with Basil, Sundried Tomatoes, and Parmesan 38

XXXII. Smoked Haddok with Lentils, Lemon, and Dill 39

XXXIII. St. David's Chicken and Leek Hotpot 41

XXXIV. Asian Noodle and Turkey Soup 42

XXXV. Speedy Tex-Mex Rice 43

XXXVI. Singapore Noodles with Chinese Cabbage and Shrimp 44

XXXVII. Juicy Lucy Pudding 46

XXXVIII. Coconut Noodle and Vegetable Soup 47

XXXIX. Mango Passion Fruit Roulade	49
XL. Poppy Seed, Parmesan, and Caraway Twists	51
XLI. Coconut Fish Sticks	52
XLII. Ricotta Lemon Pancakes	53
XLIII. Arugula Pesto	55
XLIV. Beet Greens	56
XLV. Avocado Salad	57
XLVI. Baked Salmon with Mango Avocado Salsa	58
XLIX. Sunbutter Crunch Granola	62
L. Curried Rice with Shrimp	63
LI. Pomelo Green Beans	64
Conclusion	66
Part 2	67
Introduction	68
Gluten-Free Recipes	74
Chicken roast	74
Chicken and potato curry	75
Baked fish	76
Fried mutton chops	77
Mutton and spinach curry	78
Coconut fish curry	79
Chicken kebabs	80
Beef with okra	81

Chicken fried rice 82

Shepherd's pie 84

Beef with gram pulse 85

Fried fish 87

Mixed fruit salad 88

Chicken with capsicum 89

Beef and vegetables soup 90

Sweet and sour chicken 91

Chicken with pineapples 93

Chicken ginger 94

Chicken with almond 95

Chicken and broccoli with lemon sauce 96

Chicken Manchurian 97

Chicken with orange 98

Chicken with spinach 99

Chicken jalfrezy 101

Baked chicken 102

Chicken sash lick 103

Beef with saffron rice 104

Chicken and chickpea curry 106

Chicken saffron rice 107

Chicken with garlic sauce 108

Spicy chicken with mixed vegetables 109

Egg curry	110
Eggs and vegetables fried rice	112
Scrambled spicy eggs	114
Beef with onion	115
Chicken with chilies	116
Beef with chilies	117
Chicken and potato cutlets	118
Chicken BBQ	119
Beef BBQ	120
Chicken BBQ kebabs	121
Beef BBQ kebabs	122
Beef steak	123
Chicken steak	124
Beef and gram pulses curry	125
Chicken with tomatoes	127
Minced beef with capsicum	128
Chicken with capsicum	129
Mined beef with potatoes	130
Mutton and potato curry	132
Minced beef and spinach	134
Minced beef with peas	135
Chicken, peas and potato rice	136
Chicken salad	137

Beef salad	138
Chicken and vegetables soup	139
Beef with mixed vegetables soup	140
Chicken with baby corns	141
Chicken with mushrooms	142
Beef with lentils	143
Creamy chicken pasta	144
Baked beef pasta	145
Sweet and sour spaghetti	147
Gluten-free tortillas	148
Potato tortillas	149
Corn and egg tortillas	150
Creamy tomato and egg soup	151
Chicken and mushroom soup	152
Corn and chicken rice	153
Fried chicken	154
Chicken and tomato curry	155
Chicken green curry	157
Chicken coconut curry	158
Grilled chicken with vegetables	159
Roast chicken with stir fried vegetables	160
Minced meat and potato cutlet	161
Spicy prawn rice	162

Sweet and sour prawns	163
Chicken spicy BBQ	164
Mutton BBQ chops	165
Chicken gluten-free pizza	166
Mutton grilled chops	168
Mutton roast	169
Mutton and potato curry	170
Mutton and okra curry	171
Mutton with mixed vegetables	172
Mutton spicy rice	173
Minced meat Pizza	175
Mutton BBQ	177
Mutton green coconut curry	178
Mutton jalfrezy	179
Mutton ginger	181
Mutton BBQ kebab	182
Mutton with peas	183
Mutton with capsicum	184
Mutton and almond curry	185
Conclusion	186

Part 1

Introduction

Thousands of people are shifting towards a gluten-free diet because they have heard that gluten is bad for the health, others already have allergic issues. This recipe book will help you find tasty gluten-free recipes that you and your family will love.

Thanks again for downloading this book, I hope you enjoy it!

Recipes

Grilled Marinated Shrimp

Ingredients:

- 2 pounds of large shrimp, peeled and deveined (leave the tails on)
- 1 cup of olive oil
- 3 garlic cloves minced
- ¼ cup fresh parsley, chopped
- 2 tbsps hot pepper sauce
- 1 tbsp tomato paste
- juice of 1 lemon
- 2 tsps dried oregano
- 1 tsp ground black pepper
- 1 tsp salt
- skewers (if using wooden ones, soak them in water for at least 30 minutes before using)

Directions:

1) In a bowl, mix lemon juice, olive oil, tomato paste, garlic, black pepper, oregano, hot sauce, salt, and parsley. Save some for basting purposes. In a resealable bag, pour the remaining marinade and the shrimp. Seal then place in the refrigerator to marinate for 2 hours.

2) Preheat the grill on medium-high heat. Skewer the shrimp, threading through the tail once and out near the head. Throw away the marinade.

3) Oil the grate lightly. Cook the skewered shrimp for 5 minutes on each side, basting it from time to time with the reserved marinade.

4) This makes 6 servings.

II. **Barbecued Beef**

Ingredients:

- 4 pounds chuck roast (boneless)
- ¼ cup of red wine vinegar
- 1 ½ cups of ketchup
- 2 tbsps Dijon-style mustard
- ¼ cup brown sugar, packed
- 2 tbsps Worcestershire sauce
- ¼ tsp garlic powder
- ¼ tsp black pepper, ground
- 1 tsp liquid smoke flavoring
- ½ tsp salt

Directions:

1) In a big bowl, combine red wine vinegar, brown sugar, liquid smoke, Dijon-style mustard, ketchup, and Worcestershire sauce. Add in the garlic powder, salt, and pepper.

2) Put the chuck roast inside a slow cooker. Pour in the sauce over the mixture. Cover the cooker and leave to cook on low setting for 8-10 hours.

3) Take out the roast from the cooker, and using a fork, shred the meat. Return the shredded roast to the cooker. Stir well in order for the sauce to cover everything. Continue cooking the roast for about another hour.

4) This makes 12 servings.

III.Baked Kale Chips

Ingredients:

- A bunch of kale
- 1 tablespoon of olive oil

Directions:

1) Preheat the oven to 350 degrees Fahrenheit. Line a cookie sheet (non-insulated) with parchment paper.

2) Using kitchen shears or a knife, carefully take out the leaves from the stems. Tear the leaves into bite-sized pieces. Wash the pieces well then dry thoroughly using a salad spinner.

3) Drizzle the kale with the olive oil then season with some salt for taste.

4) Bake the leaves until the edges become brown in color but are not burnt. This takes about 10-15 minutes.

5) This serves 6.

IV. Roasted Yam and Kale Salad

Ingredients:

3 tbsps olive oil

2 jewel yams, cut into cubes (about 1-inch)

1 onion, sliced

3 garlic cloves, minced

2 tbsps red wine vinegar

1 bunch kale, torn into pieces (bite-sized)

1 tsp fresh thyme, chopped

Salt and black pepper (freshly ground) to taste

Directions:

1) Preheat the oven to 400 degrees Fahrenheit. In a bowl, toss the yams with 2 tbsps of the olive oil. Season with salt and pepper to taste. Arrange the pieces on a baking sheet evenly.

2) Bake the yams until tender, about 20 to 25 minutes. Take out from the oven then leave to cool to room temperature inside the refrigerator.

3) In a large skillet on medium heat, heat the remaining 1 tbsp olive oil. Saute the garlic and the onion until onion caramelizes and turns golden brown. This takes about 15 minutes. Add in the kale and cook until it is wilted and tender. Transfer the kale into a bowl, and put in the refrigerator to cool to room temperature.

4) Once everything has cooled, combine the red wine vinegar, yams, fresh thyme, and kale in a bowl. Season with salt and pepper to taste then stir gently to combine.

V. Black Beans and Quinoa

Ingredients:

- 1 tsp vegetable oil
- 2 cans (15-ounces each) black beans, rinsed and then drained
- 1 onion, chopped
- ¾ cup quinoa (uncooked)
- 3 garlic cloves, peeled then chopped
- 1 ½ cups of vegetable broth
- ¼ tsp cayenne pepper
- ½ cup fresh cilantro, chopped
- 1 cup corn kernels (frozen)
- 1 tsp ground cumin
- Salt and pepper to taste

Directions:

1) In a medium saucepan, heat the oil over medium heat. Saute the garlic and onion until they are lightly browned.

2) Add in the quinoa to the saucepan and the vegetable broth. Season with cayenne pepper, cumin, pepper, and salt. Bring everything to a boil. Cover, lower the heat, and leave to simmer for 20 minutes.

3) Stir in the frozen corn into the mixture, and leave to simmer for 5 minutes more. The corn should be fully

heated through. Add in the cilantro and the black beans.

4) This makes 10 servings

VI. **Caramel Pork Chops**

Ingredients:

- 4 thick pork chops (about ¾ of an inch thick)
- 2 tart apples, cored, peeled, and sliced
- 1 tsp vegetable oil
- 1/8 tsp ground cinnamon
- 1/8 tsp ground nutmeg
- 2 tbsps brown sugar
- 2 tbsps unsalted butter
- 3 tbsps pecans
- Salt and pepper to taste

Directions:

1) Preheat the oven to 175 degrees Fahrenheit. Place an oven-proof medium-sized dish inside the oven to warm it.

2) On medium-high heat, heat a large skillet. Brush both sides of the pork chops lightly with oil. Cook the pork for 5 to 6 minutes, turning occasionally or

until they are done. Transfer the chops onto the warm dish. Keep them warm inside the preheated oven.

3) Inside a small bowl, combine the cinnamon, nutmeg, brown sugar, salt, and pepper. Inside the same skillet where the chops were cooked, add in butter then the apples and sugar mixture. Cover the mixture and cook until the apples are tender. With a slotted spoon, remove the apples and place on top of the pork chops. Keep the chops warm inside the oven.

4) Continue cooking the sauce without any cover until it becomes slightly thickened. Spoon the sauce over the chops and apples. Sprinkle the top with pecans.

5) This makes 4 servings.

VII. Roasted Brussels Sprouts

Ingredients:

- 1 ½ lbs Brussels sprouts with the yellow leaves removed and the ends trimmed
- 1 tsp kosher salt
- 3 tbsps olive oil
- ½ tsp black pepper (freshly ground)

Directions:

1) Preheat the oven to 400 degrees Fahrenheit.

2) Place the Brussels sprouts, kosher salt, olive oil, and pepper inside a big zip-lock plastic bag. Seal the plastic tightly and shake well to coat the sprouts.

3) Pour the sprouts onto a baking sheet, and put the sheet on the center oven rack.

4) Roast the Brussels sprouts in the preheated oven for 30-45 minutes. Shake the pan every 5-7 minutes so that they brown evenly. If needed, you can reduce the heat to prevent the sprouts from burning. The sprouts should be very dark brown or almost black in color when done. You can add more kosher salt if needed. Serve the sprouts immediately.

5) This makes 6 servings.

VIII. Roasted Garlic Cauliflower

Ingredients:

- 1 cauliflower head, large, separated into small florets
- 3 tbsps olive oil

- 2 tbsps minced garlic
- 1/3 cup Parmesan cheese, grated
- 1 tbsp chopped fresh parsley
- Salt and black pepper to taste

Directions:

1) Preheat the oven to 450 degrees Fahrenheit. Lightly oil or grease a big casserole dish.

2) In a resealable bag, place the garlic and olive oil. Add in the cauliflower then shake. Pour the cauliflower into the prepared dish then add salt and pepper to taste.

3) Bake the cauliflower for 25 minutes. About halfway through, stir the cauliflower. Top with parsley and Parmesan cheese and broil for 3-5 minutes until the color turns golden brown.

4) This makes 6 servings.

IX. Roasted Cauliflower Soup

Ingredients:

- 2 cauliflower heads separated into florets
- 6 cups of water
- Cooking spray (olive oil)

- 1 onion, large, chopped
- 4 cloves of garlic, chopped
- ¼ cup of olive oil
- salt and pepper (freshly ground) to taste

Directions:

1) Put the cauliflower florets in a large bowl with lightly salted water. Let the florets sit for 20 minutes then drain. Prepare a baking sheet by placing heavy aluminum foil on it. Arrange the florets on the foil and evenly spray with cooking spray.

2) Preheat the broiler of the oven and place the oven rack about 6 inches above the heat source.

3) Broil the florets until they become brown, about 20-30 minutes.

4) In a big soup pot, heat the olive oil and sauté the onion until it becomes translucent. Add in the garlic and the roasted cauliflower. Add in the water and season with black pepper and salt. Simmer until the florets become tender. Using an immersion hand blender, blend the soup inside the pot until the mixture is smooth and creamy.

5) This serves 6.

X. Buckwheat Crepes

Ingredients:

- 4 ounces of buckwheat flour
- 8 ounces of milk
- 2 tbsps coconut or olive oil
- 4 large eggs
- A pinch of kosher salt

Directions:

1) Whisk the eggs and milk together. Add in the salt and buckwheat flour. Whisk everything well.

2) Over low heat, set a big cast-iron skillet then slowly bring up the heat to medium-high. Add in some of the coconut oil. When the oil has already melted, add in some crepe batter, about 2 ounces. Tilt the skillet until the batter covers the whole surface. When the edges are already set and start curling up, flip the crepe.

3) The recipe makes 4-6 crepes, depending on how much batter you place in the skillet.

XI. Honey-Roasted Cinnamon Walnut Butter

Ingredients:

- 2 cups of shelled walnuts
- 1 tsp honey
- ¼ tsp salt
- 2 tsps walnut, canola, or grapeseed oil
- 1 tsp roasted Saigon cinnamon

Directions:

1) In a big bowl, place the walnuts and cover with water. Leave them to soak overnight. This will take out some of the bitterness.

2) Preheat the oven to 350 degrees Fahrenheit. Drain the water. On a baking sheet, spread out the walnuts in a single layer. Toast the walnuts until they are thoroughly dry and are toasted a bit. This takes about 15 minutes. Be sure to turn them about halfway through. Take the sheet out of the oven and let the walnuts cool completely.

3) In a food processor, put in the toasted walnuts. Process the walnuts until the mixture starts to become sticky. Add in the honey, salt, and cinnamon. Pulse everything then taste if the paste needs more salt, cinnamon, or honey. Keep the food processor on and slowly add in the oil.

4) This makes about a cup of walnut butter.

XII. **Weight Watchers Cabbage Soup**

Ingredients:

- 2 cups of chopped cabbage
- 3 cups of non-fat beef broth
- Half cup chopped carrots
- Half cup chopped zucchini
- Half of a yellow onion
- 2 cloves of garlic, minced
- Half cup green beans
- 1 tbsp tomato paste
- 1/2 tsp oregano
- ½ tsp basil
- Salt and pepper to taste

Directions:

1) Spray the bottom of a pot with non-stick cooking spray then sauté garlic, onions, and carrots for 5 minutes.

2) Add the cabbage, green beans, broth, tomato paste, oregano, and basil. Season with salt and pepper to taste.

3) Simmer the soup for 5-10 minutes until the vegetables become tender. Add in the zucchini, and let the soup simmer for an additional 5 minutes.

XIII. Homemade Salsa

Ingredients:

- 8 cups of tomatoes, peeled, chopped then drained
- 1 ½ cups of green peppers
- 6 cloves of garlic, minced
- 2 ½ cups of chopped onions
- 2 tsps cumin
- 2 tsps pepper
- 1 cup chopped jalapeno pepper
- 1/3 cup of sugar
- 1/3 cup of vinegar
- 1/8 cup of canning salt
- 1 can (12-ounce) tomato paste
- 1 can (15-ounce) tomato sauce

Directions:

1) Mix everything together in a saucepan and bring to a boil (slow) for about 10 minutes.

2) Transfer the salsa in jars and place in a hot water bath for 10 minutes.

3) This makes 3 to 6 quarts.

Note: If you want your salsa to be smoother, you can cut the vegetables into smaller pieces.

XIV. Roasted Broccoli with Lemon Garlic and Toasted Pine Nuts

Ingredients:

- 1 pound broccoli florets
- 2 tbsps unsalted butter
- ½ tsp grated lemon zest
- 1 to 2 tbsps lemon juice (fresh)
- 2 tbsps olive oil
- 1 tsp minced garlic
- 2 tbsps toasted pine nuts
- Salt and pepper

Directions:

1) Preheat the oven to 500 degrees Fahrenheit.

2) In a big bowl, toss the oil and broccoli. Add salt and pepper to taste.

3) On a baking sheet, arrange the florets (single layer). Roast the broccoli in the oven for 12 minutes or until the florets are just tender. Turn them once.

4) In a small saucepan on medium heat, melt the butter.

5) Add the lemon zest and garlic and heat for about a minute while stirring.

6) Let the mixture cool a bit and add in the lemon juice.

7) Put the broccoli inside a serving bowl and pour the lemon butter. Toss to coat all of the florets.

8) Scatter the pine nuts on top.

9) This serves 4.

XV. Crustless Spinach Quiche

Ingredients:

- 10 ounce package of frozen spinach (thawed)
- 1 tbsp vegetable oil
- ¾ pounds of grated muenster cheese
- 1 onion, hopped
- 5 eggs

- Salt and pepper to taste

Directions:

1) Preheat the oven to 350 degrees Fahrenheit.

2) Spray a quiche dish or 9-inch pie plate with cooking spray.

3) On medium-high heat, heat the oil in a skillet. Saute the onion until it becomes brown.

4) Add in the spinach. Cook until the extra moisture evaporates. Let it cool.

5) In a bowl, beat the eggs then add the cheese.

6) Stir the cheese and egg mixture into the spinach-onion mixture. Season with salt and pepper to taste.

7) Transfer the mixture into the pie pan and spread evenly.

8) Bake for 40-45 minutes, until the top is brown and a toothpick, when inserted at the center, comes out clean.

XVI. Oven-Dried Tomatoes

Ingredients:

- 2 tbsps extra-virgin olive oil
- Cherry tomatoes, 2 pints, cut into halves
- 2 tbsps chopped oregano
- 3 tbsps chopped basil
- 2 garlic cloves, minced
- Salt and pepper

Directions:

1) Preheat the oven to 225 degrees Fahrenheit.

2) Add oregano, olive oil, garlic, basil, salt, and pepper to the tomatoes.

3) On a cookie sheet lined with parchment paper, spread out the tomatoes and place in the oven.

4) Bake the tomatoes for an hour. Turn off the oven then let the tomatoes sit inside overnight.

5) This serves 1.

XVII. Grilled Moroccan Chicken

Ingredients:

- 4 chicken breasts, skinless and boneless
- ½ cup extra-virgin olive oil
- 2 tsps paprika

- ¼ cup chopped scallion (only the white part)
- ¼ cup fresh cilantro, chopped
- ¼ cup parsley, chopped
- 2 tsps ground cumin
- 1 tbsp minced garlic
- 1 tsp salt
- ¼ tsp cayenne pepper
- ¼ tsp turmeric

Directions:

1) Combine the parsley, scallions, oil, cilantro, paprika, garlic, salt, cumin, cayenne pepper, and turmeric in a food processor. Process until the mixture is smooth.

2) Rub the chicken with the herb mix on both sides. Let the chicken stand for 30 minutes.

3) Preheat the grill to medium heat.

4) Grill the chicken breasts for 5 to 7 minutes on each side or until the meat is fully cooked.

5) This serves 4.

XVIII. Cream of Broccoli Soup

Ingredients:

- 3 cups of roughly cut fresh broccoli
- 1 tbsp organic coconut oil or olive oil
- ¼ cup of sweet onion, diced
- 3 cups of packed stemmed greens like kale and spinach
- 1 inch of ginger, peeled and chopped
- Fresh water (quantity as needed)
- 2 garlic cloves, chopped
- Sea salt and pepper to taste
- 1 cup or more of light coconut milk
- 2 tbsps chopped mint
- 2 tbsps chopped cilantro
- 2 tbsps chopped fresh parsley

Directions:

1) In a large soup pot, heat oil over medium heat. Saute the onion, garlic, and ginger.

2) Add in the greens and broccoli. Add enough water to cover the vegetables. Don't add too much at this stage.

3) Bring the mixture to a high simmer. Cover the pot then lower the heat to medium simmer. Continue cooking until the vegetables are tender.

4) Add the chopped mint, cilantro, and parsley. Season with freshly ground pepper and sea salt.

5) Take the pot from the heat, and with an immersion blender, puree the soup.

6) Place the pot back on the stove and stir in the coconut milk. Heat the soup gently but do not boil. Taste and season again if needed.

7) Sprinkle fresh herbs on top before serving.

8) This serves 4.

XIX. Shrimp Scampi

Ingredients:

- 1 pound of shrimp, shelled then deveined
- 3 cloves of garlic, crushed
- 1/3 cup of extra virgin olive oil
- 1 tbsp lemon juice
- A pinch of red pepper flakes
- 1/3 cup dry white wine
- Salt
- 3 tbsps butter
- Flat leaf parsley, chopped (for garnish)

Directions:

1) In a large skillet, place olive oil and garlic. Cook on medium heat to infuse the oil with the garlic. Be careful that the garlic does not burn.

2) Add in the red pepper flakes. Increase the heat to medium high.

3) Add in the shrimp and season with a bit of salt. Continue cooking until the shrimp is just about done.

4) Add in wine and cook until the alcohol has been burned off (about a minute).

5) Add in the butter and lemon juice.

6) Garnish the top with parsley before serving.

7) This serves 2.

XX. Watermelon Lemonade

Ingredients:

- 4 cups of water
- 2 cans (12 ounces each) of frozen lemonade concentrate
- 3 cups of seedless watermelon, cubed

Directions:

1) In a food processor or blender, blend the watermelon on medium speed. Continue until the watermelon is smooth.

2) In a big punch bowl or large pitcher, place the water and lemonade concentrate.

3) Add in the watermelon and mix well.

4) Garnish the lemonade with more watermelon if you want.

5) This makes 12 servings.

XXI. Gluten-Free Pizza Crust

Ingredients:

- 2/3 cup of brown rice flour
- 2 tbsps powdered milk
- ½ cup of tapioca flour
- 2 tsps xanthan gum
- 1 tbsp dry yeast
- 1 tsp Italian seasoning
- ½ tsp salt
- 1 tsp unflavored gelatin
- ½ tsp agave syrup, honey, or sugar

- 2/3 cup of water with a temperature of 110 degrees Fahrenheit
- 1 tsp cider vinegar
- 1 tsp olive oil

Directions:

1) Preheat the oven to 425 degrees Fahrenheit.

2) In a medium-sized bowl, blend all of the ingredients on low speed using regular beaters. Beat everything on high speed for about 3 minutes.

3) If the mixer bounces around, it means that the dough is stiff. Add water if needed, a tablespoon at a time until the dough does not resist the beaters.

4) On a lightly greased 11x7-inch pan (for deep-dish pizza) or 12-inch pizza pan, put the mixture.

5) Sprinkle rice flour liberally on the dough. Press the dough into the pan while continuously sprinkling flour on the dough to prevent it from sticking to your hands.

6) Make the edges a bit thicker than the middle part to hold the toppings.

7) Bake the crust for 10 minutes then take it out and top with desired toppings and sauce.

8) Bake the pizza for 20-25 minutes until the top is golden brown in color.

9) This serves 6.

XXII. Marinated Olives

Ingredients:

- 2 cups of mixed olives
- 3 garlic cloves
- Peel of 1 big lemon, chopped
- Peel of 1 big orange, chopped
- 1 tsp chili flakes
- 2 rosemary sprigs
- 1 cup of olive oil

Directions:

1) Under cold water, rinse the olives quickly.

2) In a large bowl, put the lemon and orange peel, chili flakes, garlic, rosemary, and the olives.

3) In a large saucepan set on medium-high heat. Heat the olive oil but take it out of the heat before it starts to produce smoke. Pour the olive oil onto the olives.

4) Leave the olives to sit until the olive oil cools.

5) This appetizer is good for up to 8 servings.

XXIII. Sweet Potato and Pumpkin Mash

Ingredients:

- 2 lbs sweet potatoes, peeled and then cut into cubes (2-inch)
- 2 lbs pumpkin, peeled then seeded, cut into cubes (2-inch)
- 8 tbsps unsalted butter (or 1 stick)
- 4 cloves of garlic, peeled and sliced thinly
- 3-inch piece of ginger, peeled then sliced
- 3 shallots, peeled then sliced
- 5 fresh thyme sprigs (stems removed), finely chopped
- 2 sticks of cinnamon
- 1 tbsp brown sugar
- 2 cups of milk (rice or cow's milk)
- 2 cups of chicken or vegetable stock
- 1 tsp kosher salt
- 2 chive, chopped finely
- A pinch of nutmeg

Directions:

1) On medium heat, melt butter inside a deep pot. Add in the shallots, cinnamon sticks, thyme leaves, ginger, garlic, and brown sugar. Cook and stir until the sugar melts.

2) Add in the pumpkin, sweet potatoes, milk, and chicken/vegetable stock. Bring everything to a simmer. Lower the heat and cook until the pumpkin and potatoes are fork tender (about 30 minutes).

3) Drain the sweet potatoes and pumpkin, but save a cup of the liquid. Throw away the cinnamon and ginger. In a big bowl, mash the pumpkin and sweet potatoes. Pinch in the salt and nutmeg. Taste and season some more if needed. Add in some of the saved liquid and stir. Before serving, sprinkle the top with chives.

4) This serves 6.

XXIV. **Jazzed-up Hummus**

Ingredients:

- 10 oz hummus
- 1 tsp smoked paprika
- 1 tbsp fresh chives, chopped
- 1 tsp ground cumin

- 1 big lemon, juiced and zested
- ½ cup of olive oil
- Salt and pepper to taste

Directions:

1) In a food processor, add in the smoked paprika, chives, cumin, lemon juice and zest. Process the ingredients for some time until they are combined thoroughly.

2) Add in the hummus. While the processor is running, slowly add in the olive oil. When the hummus is creamy, stop processing the hummus.

3) Add in pepper and salt to taste.

XXV. Coconut Brown Rice

Ingredients:

- ½ of a 7-ounce can of coconut milk
- 2 tbsps coconut oil
- 2 cups of brown basmati rice
- 1/2 tsp kosher salt
- ½ tsp Madras curry powder
- ½ tsp powdered ginger
- Juice from a medium-sized lime

- 1 tsp cracked black pepper

Directions:

1) Soak the rice first in 4 cups of cool and fresh water. Leave it to sit for an hour or more. Some of the starch from the rice will be removed because of this. Using a large strainer, drain out the water.

2) Place rice into a rice cooker. Add in the lime juice, ginger, coconut milk, coconut oil, curry powder, pepper, and salt. Stir everything well. Add 3 ½ cups of fresh water. Stir well and close the lid. Turn the rice cooker to brown rice setting. Turn the rice cooker on.

3) Once the rice cooker signals that it the rice is cooked, you can then serve the rice.

XXVI. Roasted Pumpkin Seed Spread

Ingredients:

- 2 cups of toasted pumpkin seeds
- Juice from 1 big lemon
- About a quarter of a cup of olive oil
- 16 ounces of chickpeas
- 3 garlic cloves, peeled

- 1 tsp of smoked paprika

Directions:

1) Place the pumpkin seeds in a food processor. Turn the processor on in order to break up the seeds. As you process the seeds, add in the olive oil slowly. You will come up with a thick paste. Turn the processor off.

2) After forming a paste, add in the lemon juice. Add in the chick peas and the garlic. Turn on your processor and process it until the consistency is that of hummus. If the texture is still not to your liking, you can add in more olive oil while the processor is running.

3) Once you achieve the texture that you like, add in the smoked paprika until the paprika is incorporated fully. Transfer the spread into a container and let it stand in the refrigerator for 2 hours or so. This will allow the flavors to fully develop.

4) Eat the spread with crackers or vegetables.

-

XXVII. **Zucchini Casserole**

Ingredients:

- 6 medium-sized zucchini, sliced thinly
- 1 large tomato, chopped
- 1 medium-sized onion, chopped
- 2 cups of shredded mozzarella cheese
- 1 clove of garlic, minced
- 1 can (8-ounces) tomato sauce
- 1 tbsp olive oil
- 1 tsp Italian spices
- 1 tsp garlic salt

Directions:

1) Preheat the oven to 350 degrees Fahrenheit.

2) Heat the oil inside a big skillet. Add the garlic, onion, zucchini, and tomato. Cover and leave to cook until they achieve your desired tenderness. It takes about 10 minutes. Drain the vegetables.

3) Stir in the seasonings and tomato sauce.

4) In a baking dish (13x9 inches), put a layer of zucchini mixture then a layer of shredded cheese.

5) Continue making layers until the dish is full. The last layer should be cheese.

6) Bake the casserole for 25 minutes.

7) Top the casserole with shredded Romano or parmesan cheese if you want.

8) This makes 8 servings.

XXVIII. **Black Bean Brownies**

Ingredients:

- 1 can (15 ½ - ounce) black beans, rinsed then drained
- 4 tbsps cocoa powder
- 3 eggs
- ¾ cup of sugar
- 3 tbsps oil
- A pinch of salt
- 1 tsp vanilla

Directions:

1) Preheat the oven to 350 degrees Fahrenheit.

2) Mix all of the ingredients together in a food processor. Continue processing until everything is pureed.

3) Pour the batter into a cake pan (8x8) that has been lightly greased. Stir in some nuts or chocolate chips, or you may leave it plain.

4) Bake the brownies for about 30 minutes.

5) Let the brownies cool completely before you cut them.

6) This makes 16 brownies.

XXIX. **Flourless Peanut Butter Cookies**

Ingredients:

- 1 large egg, beaten
- 1 cup of sugar
- 1 cup of peanut butter
- 1 tsp of baking soda

Directions:

1) Grease the cookie sheets you will be using. Preheat your oven to 350 degrees Fahrenheit.

2) Beat the sugar and peanut butter together in a big bowl using an electric mixer. Continue until the mixture is smooth.

3) Add in the baking soda and beaten egg. Beat everything until well mixed.

4) Roll a teaspoon of dough into a round shape then place on a cookie sheet.

5) Place the balls an inch apart on the sheet. Flatten the balls with the tines of a fork in order to form a cross pattern.

6) Bake until the cookies are golden pale in color and puffed up. It takes about 10 minutes.

7) This makes 24 cookies.

XXX. **Stuffed Peppers**

Ingredients:

- 1 lb ground beef
- 6 green bell peppers
- ½ cup of long grain white rice (uncooked)
- 1 cup of water
- 2 8-ounce cans of tomato sauce
- ¼ tsp garlic powder
- 1 tsp Italian seasoning
- ¼ tsp onion powder
- 1 tbsp Worcestershire sauce
- Salt and pepper to taste

Directions:

1) Preheat the oven to 350 degrees Fahrenheit.

2) In a saucepan, put the rice and water. Let it boil. Lower the heat, cover, and continue cooking for 20 minutes. Over medium heat, cook the beef in a skillet until everything is browned evenly.

3) Take out the tops, membranes, and seeds of peppers. On a baking dish, arrange the peppers with the hollowed out sides facing up.

4) Mix the cooked rice, browned beef, Worcestershire sauce, a can of tomato sauce, onion powder, salt, garlic powder, and pepper in a bowl. Spoon equal amounts of the beef mixture into the hollowed peppers. In another bowl, mix the remaining tomato sauce and the Italian seasoning. Pour the sauce over the peppers.

5) Bake the peppers for an hour. Every 15 minutes, baste them with the sauce until peppers become tender.

6) This serves 6.

XXXI. Rice Noodles with Basil, Sundried Tomatoes, and Parmesan

Ingredients:

- 85 grams of sundried tomatoes (with 2 tablespoons of the oil)
- 250 grams medium rice noodles
- A large handful of basil leaves, torn into pieces
- 25 grams of parmesan, grated or shaved
- 3 cloves of garlic

Directions:

1) Prepare the noodles according to the instructions on the pack. Drain.

2) In a skillet, heat the oil and sauté the garlic and tomatoes for 3 minutes.

3) Toss in the noodles and most of the parmesan and basil. Season with salt and pepper.

4) Add the remaining basil and cheese on top.

5) This serves 4.

XXXII. Smoked Haddok with Lentils, Lemon, and Dill

Ingredients:

- 2 100-gram smoked haddock fillets

- 100 grams Puy lentils
- 300 ml of vegetable stock
- Zest from half of a lemon
- 1 small onion, chopped finely
- 1 carrot, chopped finely
- 1 stick of celery, chopped finely
- 50 grams baby spinach leaves
- 2 tablespoons of chopped dill
- 1 rounded tablespoon of half-fat crème fraiche

Directions:

1) Add the celery, onion, lentils, and carrot into a pan. Add in the vegetable stock and bring everything to a boil. Stir, lower the heat, then cover. Leave to simmer for about 20 to 25 minutes until the lentils become tender.

2) In a small bowl, mix half of the dill, lemon zest, and crème fraiche. Add a bit of seasoning. In a shallow dish, place the fish with a bit of water. Cover the dish with cling film. Microwave the fish for 4 to 6 minutes until the fish becomes easy to flake.

3) Once the lentils are done, add in the spinach until they are barely wilted. Add in the crème fraiche-dill mixture. Divide the cooked mixture between 2 plates that have been warmed then place the haddock on top. Scatter the remaining dill on top then serve.

4) This serves 2.

XXXIII. St. David's Chicken and Leek Hotpot

Ingredients:

- 4 chicken breasts, diced (skinless and boneless)
- 2 red potatoes, peeled then cut into chunks
- 3 medium-sized carrots, peeled then cut into 1 ¼-inch slices
- 2 leeks, washed and sliced thickly
- 300 ml of hot chicken stock
- 1 tablespoon chopped fresh parsley
- 3 tablespoons double cream

Directions:

1) In a shallow microwaveable dish, toss the carrots, potatoes, and leeks with some pepper and salt. Pour in the stock. Cover the dish using cling film and poke some holes on the film with the tip of a knife. Cook the vegetables for 10 minutes on high. The potatoes should start becoming tender.

2) Take out the dish from the microwave, remove the cling film, then add in the chicken. Cover the dish once again with fresh film and pierce with a knife again. Cook the mixture for 6 minutes on high. The chicken should be succulent and cooked by then.

3) Uncover the dish, stir in the parsley and cream, and add black pepper to taste. Serve with gluten-free bread to mop up the juices at the bottom of the dish. This serves 4.

XXXIV. Asian Noodle and Turkey Soup

Ingredients:

- 200 grams of dried rice noodles (any type will do)
- 1 ½ pounds of chicken or turkey stock
- 100 grams of bean sprouts
- 400 grams of shredded roasted turkey
- 2 star anise
- 3 cloves
- A thumb-sized piece of root ginger, peeled then sliced
- 1 cinnamon stick
- 2 limes, one sliced for wedges, the other one juiced
- 4 spring onions, sliced thinly
- 2 to 3 tablespoons of fish sauce

- 2 red chilies, sliced

- A bunch of coriander

- A bunch of mint

Directions:

1) In a big pan, pour in the stock and add in the spices and ginger. Leave the stock to simmer for 10 minutes. Soak noodles according to the package instructions. Rinse and drain.

2) Add in the lime juice and fish sauce to the stock. Taste test and add more fish sauce if needed. Divide the noodles between 4 bowls. Top noodles with beansprouts, herbs, shredded turkey, chilies, and spring onion. Ladle the hot stock onto the noodles. Serve with lime wedges and more herbs.

3) This serves 4.

XXXV. Speedy Tex-Mex Rice

Ingredients:

- 200 grams of rice

- 1 to 2 tablespoons of fajita seasoning mix or Cajun seasoning

- Juice from 1 lime

- 1 small jar of roasted peppers in olive oil, sliced (keep 3 tablespoons of the oil)

- a small bunch of coriander, chopped roughly

- 1 400-gram tin of black-eyed beans, rinsed then drained

Directions:

1) Cook the rice according to package instructions then drain. In a frying pan, heat 1 tablespoon of oil. Add in the fajita seasoning and sliced peppers. Cook for 1 minute until the mixture becomes fragrant.

2) Stir in the beans and rice. Heat until very hot. Add in the remaining oil, coriander, seasoning, and lime juice. Add some seasoning if needed then serve

3) This serves 4.

XXXVI. Singapore Noodles with Chinese Cabbage and Shrimp

Ingredients:

- 200 grams of dried rice vermicelli
- 1 Chinese cabbage, cut into slices (about 1-cm thick)
- 1 carrot sliced very thinly
- 150 ml of hot chicken stock
- 1-2 tablespoons of sunflower oil
- 1 teaspoon brown sugar
- 1 teaspoon chopped ginger
- 1 tablespoon hot curry powder
- 2 teaspoons of vinegar (any gluten-free type)
- 140 grams of bean sprouts
- 400 grams of small, cooked, and peeled prawns
- A bunch of spring onion, sliced thinly
- Soy sauce to serve
- Oriental chili oil (the one that has shrimp paste), to serve

Directions:

1) In a heatproof bowl, place the dried noodles and pour boiling water let it soak for 5 minutes or check the pack instructions. Drain it well.

2) In a wok, heat the oil then stir fry the ginger for a minute. Add in the curry powder and cook for another minute.

3) Add in the carrot and cabbage. Stir-fry for 2 more minutes. Add in the stock, vinegar, sugar, bean sprouts, prawns, and drained noodles. Cook until the mixture is piping hot. Add in the spring onions. Divide the noodles and soup between bowls. Add in soy sauce and some chili oil.

4) This serves 4.

XXXVII. Juicy Lucy Pudding

Ingredients:

· 50 grams gluten-free breadcrumbs

· 350 gram packet of frozen forest fruits, defrosted

· 6 medium-sized pears (ripe), peeled, cored, then quartered

- 4 tablespoons of wild blueberries jam (no added sugar)

- 3 tablespoons light muscovado sugar

- 25 grams melted butter

Directions:

1) Preheat the oven to 190 degrees Celsius.

2) In a big bowl, mix the forest fruits, jam, sugar, and pears. Place them inside a deep baking dish (18x28 cm). Cover the dish with foil, roast it in the oven for about 20 minutes. Check the pear if tender; if not, return the dish to the oven for 5 more minutes.

3) Mix the butter and breadcrumbs. Scatter them over the fruit. Bake again for 10-15 minutes until the breadcrumbs are crispy and golden. Serve the pudding hot.

4) This serves 4-6.

XXXVIII. Coconut Noodle and Vegetable Soup

Ingredients:

- 200 grams thick rice noodles

- 1-2 tablespoons of Thai green curry paste

- 300 ml coconut milk (reduced fat)

- 1 teaspoon ground nut oil

- 200 grams sliced chestnut mushrooms

- 700 ml vegetable stock

- 1 ½ tablespoons Thai fish sauce

- 140 grams halved sugar snap peas

- 100 grams beansprouts

- 3 shredded spring onions

- Juice from 1 lime

- A few coriander and mint leaves (to serve)

Directions:

1) Over medium heat, heat a large pan. Heat the oil and cook the Thai green curry paste for a minute. The paste should release the aroma. Pour in the coconut milk and stock and bring to a boil. Lower the heat to a simmer.

2) Stir in noodles. Let the mixture simmer for 7 minutes, then add in sugar snaps and mushrooms. Cook for another 3 minutes. Add in fish sauce, lime

juice, and beansprouts. Take the pan out of the heat.

3) Ladle the soup and noodles into bowls. Add spring onions, coriander, and mint to serve.

4) This serves 4.

XXXIX. Mango Passion Fruit Roulade

Ingredients:

· 175 grams caster sugar

· 3 big egg whites

· 4 passion fruits (pulp part)

· 1 level teaspoon of corn flour

· 1 teaspoon vanilla extract

· 1 teaspoon malt vinegar (gluten-free)

· 1 big ripe mango, peeled, seed removed, diced

· 200 grams of Greek yogurt (fat-free)

· Raspberry sauce

· Icing sugar

Directions:

1) Preheat the oven to 150 degrees Celsius. Line a Swiss roll tin (33x23 cm) with nonstick baking parchment paper. Beat the egg whites using an electric whisk until they are frothy and double in size. Slowly add in caster sugar until the mixture is shiny and thick. Mix the vinegar, vanilla extract, and cornflour then add into the egg whites.

2) Spoon the mixture into the tin and level the white carefully. Bake this for about 30 minutes until the surface of the meringue is just firm.

3) Take the meringue out of the oven then cover with a damp greaseproof paper for about 10 minutes. Take another greaseproof paper and dust with icing sugar. Discard the damp greaseproof paper, turn out the meringue on the sugarcoated paper. Peel the lining paper, then spread the yogurt on the meringue and scatter the passion fruit and mango.

4) Roll up the roulade using the paper from one of the short ends. Keep the place where the roll ends underneath. Sift some icing sugar on the top of the roll. Serve it with raspberry sauce.

5) This makes 6 servings.

XL. Poppy Seed, Parmesan, and Caraway Twists

Ingredients:

- 1 beaten egg
- 175 grams of gluten-free flour
- 1 egg yolk mixed together with 3 tablespoons of cold water
- 85 grams of butter
- A pinch of cayenne pepper
- 1 tablespoon each of caraway seeds and poppy seeds
- 3 tablespoons parmesan cheese, freshly grated

Directions:

1) In a food processor, put the butter, flour, and cayenne pepper. Process until they resemble fine breadcrumbs. Add in the egg + water mixture and pulse once again. The mixture should come together. Transfer the mixture on a board and squeeze the pastry gently until it forms a ball. Add more water if it is a bit dry.

2) Heat the oven to 190 degrees Celsius. Roll pastry into a big rectangle (about A4-size). Brush the rectangle with the beaten egg. Half the rectangle widthways. Sprinkle a half with Parmesan and the other half with the caraway and poppy seeds. Run a rolling pin lightly across the top in order to press the seeds and cheese.

3) Cut the halves into sticks (about 12-15 each). Arrange the sticks on a baking sheet then chill for about 10 minutes. After 10 minutes, bake the sticks for 8-10 minutes then leave to cool for 5 minutes. Transfer to a wire rack after 5 minutes.

4) This makes 24-30 sticks.

-

XLI. Coconut Fish Sticks

Ingredients:

· 1 ½ lbs of tilapia filets

· ½ cup of mayonnaise

· 1 large egg

· ¼ cup + 1 tsp of gluten-free tamari

· 2 ½ cups of coconut flakes

Directions:

1) Preheat the oven to 400 degrees. Position the oven racks on the bottom and top third of the oven. Using foil, line 2 baking sheets. Spray the top generously with non-stick cooking spray.

2) Take the filets and them in half lengthwise down at the center. Halve the half once again lengthwise then cut again in half crosswise.

3) In a shallow bowl, beat the egg then add the teaspoon of gluten-free tamari. On a plate, put the coconut flakes. Dip the fish into the egg, shake the excess then dip into the coconut. Press well to make the coconut flakes stick. Place the fish on the prepared baking sheets then lightly spray with cooking spray.

4) Bake the fish until they are golden brown and when they are firm to touch, about 15 to 20 minutes. Rotate the baking sheets from bottom to top halfway through.

5) Mix the gluten-free tamari and mayonnaise. Serve the sauce with the fish. This serves 4.

XLII. **Ricotta Lemon Pancakes**

Ingredients:

- Finely grated zest of a lemon
- 8 ounces of Ricotta cheese in room temperature
- 4 eggs, separated
- A big pinch of salt

Directions:

1) Beat the egg whites until stiff peaks start to form.

2) In another bowl, beat the cheese until it become creamy and smooth. Add in the yolks, salt, and lemon zest. Beat until the cheese becomes fluffy and smooth. Get about a scoop of the egg whites and mix it into the yolk mixture. After mixing it, fold in all of the remaining yolk mixture into the egg whites.

3) Heat a skillet or griddle on medium heat until it is hot. Spray it with gluten-free cooking spray.

4) Get about a third cup of the mixture and put onto the griddle. Push down the batter as it can be fluffy. Cook on medium heat until they are browned. Flip over and continue cooking. This makes 12 pancakes.

XLIII. Arugula Pesto

Ingredients:

- 2 cups of packed arugula leaves with the stems removed
- ½ of a garlic clove, peeled then minced
- ½ cup of extra virgin olive oil
- ½ cup of shelled walnuts
- ½ tsp salt
- 6 cloves of garlic, unpeeled
- ½ cup of fresh Parmesan cheese

Directions:

1) Brown the 6 cloves of garlic on a skillet on medium heat. Keep the peels on. Heat until some places are lightly browned, and this takes about 10 minutes. Take out the garlic from the pan, leave to cool, then take out the skins.

2) In a pan set over medium heat, toast the nuts until they become lightly brown.

3) In a food processor, combine the raw and roasted garlic, salt, arugula, and walnuts. Pulse everything

then slowly drizzle in the olive oil. Take out the mixture from the processor and transfer into a bowl. Stir in the Parmesan cheese.

XLIV. Beet Greens

Ingredients:

- 1 pound of beet greens
- 1 tablespoon of bacon fat or a strip of thick-cut bacon (chopped)
- 1 large clove of garlic, minced
- ¾ cup of water
- ¼ cup of chopped onion
- 1 tablespoon of granulated sugar
- 1/6 cup of cider vinegar
- ¼ teaspoon of crushed red pepper flakes

Directions:

1) Wash the beet greens in cold water. Drain then wash again. Drain and take out the heavy stems.

Tear the pieces into bite-sized pieces. Set these aside.

2) In a 3-quart saucepan or large skillet, heat the bacon fat or cook the bacon until it is lightly browned. Add the onions and cook for 5-7 minutes on medium heat. Stir it occasionally. Onions should start to brown and become soft. Add in the garlic. Add in water and stir to loosen particles that are stuck at the bottom of the pan. Stir in the red pepper and sugar. Bring the mixture to a boil.

3) Add in the beet greens then gently toss the onion mixture so the greens are well coated. Decrease the heat then cover the pan. Let the mixture simmer for 5 to 15 minutes until the greens become tender. Add in the vinegar.

4) This makes 4 servings.

XLV. **Avocado Salad**

Ingredients:

· 1 to 2 ripe avocados, seeded and quartered

· 2 tsps of fresh oregano

· 5 tablespoons of extra-virgin olive oil

- ¼ cup of chopped toasted hazelnuts
- 2 cups of cooked lentils
- 1 tbsp of fresh lemon juice
- ½ tsp of sea salt
- ¼ cup of minced chives

Directions:

1) Using a mortar and pestle, smash the salt and oregano to form a paste. Gradually add in the olive oil then the lemon juice.

2) In a bowl, toss the oregano oil and lentils. Taste and then season some more if needed. Arrange the lentils in a bowl or platter. Just before serving, quarter the avocados then slice thinly. Arrange the avocados on top of the lentils. Drizzle the salad with more oil then sprinkle with chives and hazelnuts.

3) This serves 4.

XLVI. Baked Salmon with Mango Avocado Salsa

Ingredients:

- 4 salmon fillets (6-ounces each)

- Olive oil

- 2 just ripe avocados

- 1 large or 2 small mangos

- ¼ cup of minced red onion

- Juice from 2 limes

- Freshly ground black pepper

    - Salt

- 1 serrano chili, minced

Directions:

1) Preheat the oven to 400 degrees Fahrenheit. While you are preheating the oven, prepare the mangoes. Cut them into 1/3 inch cubes (take out the seed).

2) Using aluminum foil, line a roasting pan. Put some olive oil on the foil. Coat the fillets with olive oil and lay on the foil skin side down. Sprinkle the top with salt. Bake this for 10 minutes.

3) While baking the fish, prepare the avocados. Half the avocados and take out the seeds. Using a small knife, score the inner part of the avocados, make cross hatch pattern. Scoop out the avocado and add

them in the bowl with the mango. Add the Serrano chili, minced red onion, and lime juice. Sprinkle with a bit of salt. Mix gently.

4) Serve the fillets together with the salsa. This makes 4 servings.

-

XLVII. **Mung Bean Hummus**

Ingredients:

- 1 ½ cups of cooked mung beans
- ½ cup of tahini paste
- 1 big garlic clove, peeled then smashed
- 2 tbsps of lemon juice
- ½ tsp fine grain sea salt
- 1/3 cup of water
- Olive oil, shallot, minced chives, or zaatar to serve

Directions:

1) In a food processor, add in mung beans. Pulse until a fluffy and fine crumb develops. Scrape the sides from time to time.

2) Add in the tahini, sea salt, garlic, and lemon juice. Blend once again.

3) Once you see that the beans start to form a ball, slowly add in water from time to time. Stop adding when the hummus is light, smooth, and creamy. Add more salt or lemon juice if needed.

4) This makes about 2 cups.

XLVIII. **Sticky Wings**

Ingredients:

- ½ cup of honey

- 3 lbs of chicken wings

- ½ cup of teriyaki sauce

- 2 tsps of toasted sesame seeds

Directions:

1) Preheat the oven to 475 degrees Fahrenheit. Line with foil 2 rimmed baking sheets.

2) Combine the honey and teriyaki sauce. Put half of the mixture inside a large mixing bowl. Toss in the chicken wings to coat well. Put the coated chicken wings on the baking sheets, with the skin side down.

Bake for 20 minutes. Discard if there is any leftover marinade.

3) Take 2 tablespoons from the remaining honey and teriyaki mixture and set aside. Transfer the remaining sauce in a small serving bowl. Turn the wings over, brush the 2 tablespoons and cook for 2 more minutes. Sprinkle sesame seeds on the wings and serve with the dipping sauce.

4) This serves 8.

XLIX. **Sunbutter Crunch Granola**

Ingredients:

- ¼ cup of honey
- ¼ cup of Sunbutter (creamy)
- 2 cups of gluten-free rolled oats
- ½ tsp kosher salt
- 2 tsps pure vanilla extract

Directions:

1) Preheat the oven to 325 degrees Fahrenheit. Using nonstick cooking spray, spray a cookie sheet.

2) In a microwave safe bowl, combine the honey and Sunbutter. Microwave it for 30 seconds or till the Sunbutter has already melted.

3) Stir in the oats, vanilla, and salt. Mix well to coat all of the oats. Transfer the mixture onto the cookie sheet and spread it evenly. Bake the granola for 20 minutes, stir it 1-2 times while baking.

4) Let the mixture cool. It will become crunchy when it is cooled.

5) This makes 8 – ¼ cup servings.

L. Curried Rice with Shrimp

Ingredients:

- 1 ½ pounds of large shrimp, peeled and deveined
- 2 ½ cups of water
- 1 cup of long grain white rice
- 1 tbsp olive oil
- 2 carrots, chopped
- 2 tsps curry powder
- 1 big onion, chopped
- ½ cup of fresh basil
- 2 garlic cloves, chopped
- Kosher salt and black pepper

Directions:

1) On medium heat, heat the oil inside a large skillet. Add the carrots and onion and cook for 6-8 minutes. Stir occasionally until the onion and carrots are soft.

2) Add the curry powder and garlic, and cook for 2 minutes until fragrant.

3) Add 2 ½ cups of water, rice, ½ teaspoon each of pepper and salt. Bring everything to a boil. Decrease the heat and let it simmer with a cover for 15 minutes.

4) Take ¼ tsp pepper and ½ tsp salt and season the shrimp. Place them carefully into the partially cooked rice. Cover and continue cooking until the shrimp become opaque, about 4-5 minutes. Slowly add in the basil.

5) This serves 4.

LI. **Pomelo Green Beans**

Ingredients:

- 1 lb green beans, trimmed
- 6 medium garlic cloves, peeled
- ¼ tsp of sea salt (fine grain)

- 3 to 4 tbsps extra-virgin olive oil
- ½ cup of toasted walnut halves
- 1 tbsp fresh herbs (chives, oregano, etc.)
- 1 small head radicchio, shredded finely
- 1 cup of orange or pomelo segments

Directions:

1) Boil a big pot of water and add salt. Cook the cloves of garlic for 10 minutes. Take them out with a slotted spoon or strainer. Transfer to a mortar and pestle.

2) Mash the garlic with the salt, walnut halves, and herbs. This will help make a paste. Slowly add in the olive oil until you like the consistency. Taste, then adjust if it needs more salt.

3) Add in the green beans until they become bright in color. They should be a little tender but still with good structure. Drain then put into a serving bowl. Toss the beans with the walnut-garlic dressing, then add in the radicchio, some more walnuts, and pomelo. Toss quickly then serve. This serves 4.

Conclusion

Thank you again for downloading this book!

You will certainly love the recipes that have been included in this book. There is no more need for you to stick to unhealthy gluten-stuffed food because there are a lot of other better an healthier alternatives that will not harm you and your loved ones. These recipes are all delicious and will surely make you crave for more!

Part 2

Introduction

This book contains recipes and explanation of how Gluten Free food can benefit your overall health

This e-book will help you in understanding the Benefits of going Gluten free. Gluten Free helps in treat celiac disease as gluten is being considered to be the source and cause of inflammation in the small intestineand this book will take you through different recipes that will help you to enjoy your Gluten free Journey.

Thanks again for downloading this book, I hope you enjoy it!

What is Gluten-Free Diet?

A gluten-free diet is a diet that is free of all sources of gluten protein. Sources of gluten may include wheat, rye, barley and triticale. This diet is mainly used to treat celiac disease as gluten is being considered to be the source and cause of inflammation in the small intestine. A gluten-free diet has been found to be helpful in the prevention of complications and controlling signs and symptoms associated with this disease.

Majority of all the available wide variety of foods sources do not contain gluten. Therefore diet planning and adaptation need not be difficult to achieve. Basically this diet has been a part of a treatment regimen for celiac disease. Switching to a gluten free diet is not at all that difficult as only few sources of food needed to be avoided in this. Most of the food items are gluten-free naturally and therefore a wide variety of delicious food items are available to be enjoyed in a wide variety of ways.

All natural sources of beans, nuts, seeds, eggs, meat, fish, poultry, dairy, fruits, vegetables and many grains could be enjoyed. Most of the grains and starch groups are naturally free of gluten protein which may include flax, rice, soy, corn, potato, arrowroot, amaranth, buckwheat, millet, quinoa, sorghum, tapioca, teff, etc. Foods that need to be avoided may include bulgur, farina, durum flour, Graham flour, semolina, spelt, etc. Foods that may contain gluten may include cereals, candies, cakes, pies, breads, beer, croutons, cookies, crackers, French fries, gravies, imitation meat, pastas, salad dressings, soy sauce, sauces, dips, and all processed food products.

Due to gluten intolerance or sensitivity people may choose to go for gluten-free diet. For the general public there is no solid published evidence that supports and suggests that going gluten free is helpful for them. In recent past there has been great interest in gluten-free diet in the general public and consequently the market for gluten-free food products had been expanding progressively. Majority of the people opting for a gluten-free diet had been doing so to find relief from gluten intolerance, sensitivity or allergy.

A word of caution is needed here as unnecessary use of this diet may lead towards food nutrient deficiencies. Wheat flour contains around 12% gluten. Many people consider a gluten-free diet a fad but still there are many who believe that cutting down on many sources of gluten is benefitting them. Gluten-free products have been progressively gaining strength on shelves of super markets and grocery stores. Many people who are not even fully aware of how many benefits this diet has to offer this diet has been part of their dietary trend.

Gluten is a plant protein found mainly in wheat, rye and barley and all food products that contains these food items and helps in maintaining the elasticity of foods during the fermentation phase of food production. It is due to the presence of gluten in bread that we find it chewy. As refined flour is mixed with water it gets more and more elastic during kneading process and this is due to the presence of gluten protein.

Benefits of Gluten-Free Diet

Basically a gluten-free diet has a lot to offer if you are suffering from celiac disease, are hypersensitive to gluten or are diagnosed with gluten intolerance. Opting for a gluten free diet may indirectly help you in eliminating many unhealthy food items and food products from your diet that otherwise you are unable to do so e. g. cakes, pastries, cookies, dough nuts and many creamy high in saturated fat and trans-fats food sources of food products. Pure chocolate is gluten free.

But as we are aware that the market for alternatives for gluten-free food products is expanding explosively, this particular protective beneficial element attached with it may get eliminated in due time. If someone is getting benefitted by not eating pastries and cakes today tomorrow they may find gluten-free sources of the same and therefore this beneficial aspect of it will wipe out with time as more gluten-free commercial products starts appearing in the market.

Commercially prepared food products should be avoided in all circumstances because these ontain artificial colors, chemicals and preservatives. Synthetic ingredients have negative effects on overall health and well-being. Consuming a gluten-free diet may help in promoting weight loss if taken in a well-planned and well-balanced manner. For good health benefits, right food items needed to be taken in right proportion.

Keep portion size in mind and be sure to add gluten free starch sources of food items such as sweet potatoes, potatoes, rice, quinoa, corn, etc. Going gluten free may mean saying no to many healthy and nutritious sources of food. Until and unless you are diagnosed with celiac disease or sure of being allergic, sensitive or intolerant to gluten protein you may need not follow this diet as doing so may lead to food nutrient deficiencies.

Gluten rich food sources are also rich sources of many nutrients and cutting down on these foods may mean cutting down on many nutrients. Good dietary planning is needed in order to furnish all the essential nutrients in required quantity on a daily basis to avoid food deficiencies. Meeting the dietary guidelines is a challenge while following this diet.

When you are following a gluten free diet, try to eat home cooked meals instead of eating out. Many gluten free products are available at specialty retailers. Oats can be consumed in moderate amount although these might have been cross contaminated during harvesting or processing. Gluten free bread can be made from other sources of starch which may include rice flour, potato flour, sorghum flour, corn flour, legumes flour, beans flour, almond flour, etc. These flour do not form elasticity during kneading and therefore guar gum, xantham gum, hydroxypropyle methylcellulose, eggs, corn starch may needed to be added to compensate for gluten protein. These may be helpful in retaining the shape and make bread fluffier.

Gluten is generally regarded as safe and therefore food products containing this may not be notified through systematic labeling procedure. People with gluten sensitivity are unable to metabolize gluten properly and this results in digestive distress. Symptoms of digestive distress may include gas, bloating, diarrhea, constipation or bowel discomfort.

Gluten sensitivity is less severe and digestive symptoms may occur after the intake of gluten and does not appear to have long term effects. A gluten free diet or gluten reduced diet is suggested to prevent the discomfort. There has been misunderstanding among the general public as this diet is being presumed to show a patterns of healthy eating guidelines. It does, but only for the ones who are showing signs and symptoms of gluten sensitivity and not for the general public.

Gluten-Free Recipes

Chicken roast

Ingredients

Chicken quarters 4
Ginger and garlic paste 3 table spoons
Unsweetened yogurt ½ cup
Vinegar ¼ cup
Green chili paste 2 table spoons
Salt and pepper to taste
Sesame seeds oil ¼ cup

Directions

1. Mix all the ingredients well together and refrigerate for few hours for marinating.
2. Pre-heat oven at medium heat and roast it till it gets tender and attain right color.
3. Serve hot with gluten free sauces and dips of choice.

Chicken and potato curry

Ingredients

Chicken with bones small pieces 1 lb.
Potatoes 2 cut in quarters
Onion 3 finely sliced and fried golden brown
Yogurt 1 cup
Red chili powder 1 tea spoon
Ginger and garlic paste 3 table spoons
Coriander seeds powder 1 tea spoon
Cumin seeds powder 1 tea spoon
Five spice powder ½ tea spoon
Green chilies whole 3
Coriander leaves ½ cup chopped
Salt to taste
Oil ½ cup

Directions

1. Blend fried onion and yogurt together.
2. Heat oil in a sauce pan and fry chicken with ginger and garlic paste.
3. Add blended ingredients and all the ingredients except coriander leaves.
4. Add four cups of water and bring to boil.
5. Simmer, cover and cook till potatoes and chicken get tender.

6. Remove from stove and add chopped coriander leaves and serve hot with plain rice.

Baked fish

Ingredients

Fish fillet 1 lb.
Coconut cream ½ cup
Lemon juice ¼ cup
Green chili paste 2 table spoons
Salt and pepper to taste
Sesame seed oil ¼ cup

Directions

1. Mix together all the ingredients well, cover and keep refrigerated for few hours for marinating.
2. Pre heat oven at medium temperature and bake fish till it gets tender and gain required golden color.
3. Serve hot with salads and plain rice.

Fried mutton chops

Ingredients

Mutton chops 1 lb.
Ginger garlic paste 3 table spoons
Coriander seeds powder 1 tea spoon
Cumin seeds powder 1 tea spoon
Yogurt ¼ cup
Lemon juice 3 table spoon
Raw papaya paste 2 table spoon
Green chili paste 1 table spoon
Garam masala ingredients, cardamom small 4, cloves4, cardamom large 2, cinnamon 1 inch stick 1, mace 1 tea spoon, nutmeg 1/2 tea spoon, grind all the ingredients in a coffee grinder (use 1 tea spoon of the ground powder for marinating)
Salt and pepper to taste

Directions

1. Mix all the ingredients well together, cover and refrigerate for few hours for marinating.
2. Deep fry till tender.
3. Serve hot with salads and plain rice.

Mutton and spinach curry

Ingredients

Mutton leg small pieces 1 lb. wash thoroughly
Spinach 3 cups
Onion 2 sliced
Tomatoes 4 chopped
Ginger and garlic paste 3 table spoons
Cinnamon powder ¼ tea spoon
Mace powder ¼ tea spoon
Nutmeg powder ¼ tea spoon
Salt to taste
Oil ½ cup

Directions

1. Fry onion in oil till golden brown.
2. Add chopped tomatoes, ginger and garlic paste and fry.
3. Add mutton and all spices and three cups of water and bring to boil.
4. Simmer, cover and cook on low heat till mutton gets tender.
5. Add spinach and cook uncovered for few minutes.
6. Simmer and cook on low heat for five to ten minutes.
7. Serve hot with rice.

Coconut fish curry

Ingredients

Fish boneless 1 lb. 1 inch cubes
Coconut milk 1 cup
Tomato puree 1 cup
Mustard seeds 1 table spoon
Curry leaves few if available
Fenugreek seed 1 tea spoon
Ginger cloves 6 finely sliced
Salt to taste
Oil ½ cup

Directions

1. Fry fish in oil till brown, take it out in a container.
2. In the same oil fry mustard seeds, fenugreek seeds, curry leaves and garlic slice.
3. Add tomato puree, coconut milk, fried fish and salt and simmer, cover and cook for few more minutes.
4. Serve hot with plain rice.

Chicken kebabs

Ingredients

Chicken 1 lb. boneless fillet
Onion 2 cut in quarters
Ginger 1 inch piece
Garlic cloves 8
Green chilies 6
Coriander leaves ½ cup
Mint leaves ¼ cup
Lemon juice 2 table spoons
Cumin seeds 1 table spoon
Coriander seeds 1 table spoon
Salt to taste
Oil for shallow frying

Directions

1. Except oil, chop all the ingredients well in a chopper.
2. Make round disc shaped kebabs between the palms of your hand and shallow fry from both sides till done.
3. Serve hot.

Beef with okra

Ingredients

Beef ½ lb. boneless cubes
Onion 2 sliced
Tomatoes 4 chopped
Ginger and garlic paste 2 table spoons
Five spice powder or garam masala powder ½ tea spoon
Red chili powder 1 tea spoon
Okra 2 cups fried
Cumin seeds powder ½ tea spoon
Coriander seeds powder ½ tea spoon
Salt to taste
Oil ½ cup

Directions

1. Fry onion slice in oil till golden brown.
2. Add ginger and garlic paste and tomatoes and fry till mushy.
3. Add beef cubes, all spices and enough water needed to make meat tender and for curry.
4. Cover, simmer and cook on low heat till meat gets tender.
5. Add fried okra and cook for few more minutes.
6. Serve hot with rice.

Chicken fried rice

Ingredients

Chicken ½ lb. boneless cubes
Mixed vegetables 3 cups, julienne, carrots, onion, capsicum, spring onion, cabbage
Garlic cloves 8 sliced
Rice 2 cups, long grain basmati, wash and soak for half an hour
Soy sauce ½ cup gluten free
Salt to taste
Oil ½ cup

Directions

1. Fry garlic slices in half oil till golden brown.
2. Add chicken cubes and fry till tender.
3. Add vegetable, salt and half soy sauce and fry.
4. Strain out excess water from rice.
5. Add rice and three cups of boiling water, remaining soy sauce, oil and two tea spoons salt and bring to boil.
6. Cover and cook on medium heat till all the water dries.
7. Keep it over pre heated skillet for five to ten more minutes.

8. Uncover rice pan and add fried chicken and vegetables and mix well.
9. Serve hot.

Shepherd's pie

Ingredients

Potatoes 3 boiled and mashed
Beef minced 1 lb.
Onion 2 chopped
Green chilies 3 chopped
Ginger and garlic paste 2 table spoons
Butter 3 table spoon
Milk 1 cup hot
Salt to taste
Black pepper to taste
Oil ¼ cup

Directions

1. Add butter, salt, pepper and warm milk in mashed potatoes and mix well
2. Fry onion in oil till it softens.
3. Add minced meat, ginger and garlic paste, green chilies, salt and pepper and fry till meat gets tender.
4. In a baking dish evenly spread a layer of mashed potatoes.
5. On top of this layer add minced meat layer.
6. Bake at medium heat in a pre-heated oven for 15-20 minutes or till done.
7. Serve hot.

Beef with gram pulse

Ingredients

Beef 1 lb. boneless cubes
Gram pulses 1 cup wash and soak for one hour
Onion 2 sliced
Garlic and ginger paste 3 table spoons
Tomatoes 4 chopped
Cumin seeds powder 1 tea spoon
Coriander seeds powder 1 tea spoon
Red chili powder 1 tea spoon
Turmeric powder ½ tea spoon
Five spice mix or garam masala powder ½ tea spoon
Coriander leaves ½ cup chopped
Salt to taste
Oil ½ cup

Directions

1. Fry onion in oil till golden brown.
2. Add tomatoes and ginger and garlic paste and cook till it becomes mushy.
3. Add beef, gram pulse and all the spices and enough water for beef and gram pulse to get tender.
4. Mix well, cover, simmer and cook till meat and gram pulse get tender.

5. Garnish with freshly chopped coriander leaves and enjoy with plain rice.

Fried fish

Ingredients

Fish fillet 1 lb.
Soy sauce 2 table spoons gluten free
Ginger paste 2 table spoons
Lemon juice 3 table spoons
Coconut cream powder 1 table spoon
3 table spoons
Green chili paste 2 table spoons
Salt to taste
Oil for shallow frying

Directions

1. Mix all the ingredients well except oil and marinate fish in the refrigerator for few hours.
2. Shallow fry it from both sides and serve hot with plain rice.

Mixed fruit salad

Ingredients

Apple 1 diced
Banana 1 sliced
Orange 1 sliced
Pear 1 diced
Papaya 1 cup diced
Lemon juice 3 table spoons
Molasses 3 table spoons
Cinnamon powder 1/4 tea spoon

Directions

1. Mix all the ingredients well and serve cold.

Chicken with capsicum

Ingredients

Chicken 1 lb. small pieces with bones
Capsicum 1 cup diced
Tomatoes 4 chopped
Onion 2 sliced
Ginger and garlic paste 2 table spoons
Five spice mix or garam masala ½ tea spoon
Red chili powder 1 tea spoon
Cumin seeds powder 1 tea spoon
Coriander powder 1 tea spoon
Salt to taste
Oil ½ cup

Directions

1. Fry onion till golden brown.
2. Add tomatoes and ginger and garlic paste 3 table spoons and fry till mushy.
3. Add chicken, all the spices and 2 cups of water and mix well. Cover, simmer and cook on low heat till chicken gets tender.
4. Add capsicum and mix well, cover, simmer and cook for five to ten more minutes.
5. Serve hot with rice.

Beef and vegetables soup

Ingredients

Beef 1cup boneless small cubes
Beef bones 2-3
Garlic 7 cloves whole
Olives 1 cup whole
Mushrooms 1 cup whole
Avocado 1 whole
Onion 1 whole
Tomatoes 4 whole
Coriander leaves 1 cup
Salt and black pepper to taste
Olive oil 3 table spoons

Directions

1. Boil beef with bones and without bones together in enough water, simmer, cover and cook on low heat till beef gets tender.
2. Mix all the vegetables together and bring to boil, simmer, cover and cook till vegetables get tender.
3. Blend all the vegetables in a blender.
4. Heat oil fry boneless beef pieces till lightly brown.
5. Remove bones and add bone and beef broth to fried beef.
6. Add blended vegetables, mix well and serve hot.

Sweet and sour chicken

Ingredients

Chicken 1 cup boneless cubes
Vegetables 1/2 cup slices or cubes each, cabbage, carrots, capsicum, spring onion, onion
Tomato puree 1 cup
Soy sauce ½ cup gluten free
Corn flour ½ cup
Chicken broth 3 cups
Vinegar ¼ cup
Molasses ¼ cup
Green chili chopped 2
Garlic cloves 8 sliced
Salt to taste
Oil ½ cup

Directions

1. Fry garlic slice in ¼ cup till golden brown.
2. Add chicken cubes and fry.
3. Add vegetables and fry.
4. In a separate sauce pan fry green chilies and add molasses, vinegar, soy sauce and salt.
5. Dissolve corn flour in I cup broth and add it to the green chili sauce pan.
6. Add all the remaining broth and bring it to boil.

7. Add this sauce to stir fried vegetables and chicken and cook for one more minute on high heat.
8. Serve hot with rice.

Chicken with pineapples

Ingredients

Chicken 1 cup boneless cubes
Pineapple 1 cup cubes
Onion 1 diced
Capsicum I diced
Garlic 6 cloves sliced
Soy sauce ½ cup gluten free
Vinegar ¼ cup
Chicken broth 1 cup
Corn flour ¼ cup
Salt to taste
Oil ½ cup

Directions

1. Fry garlic slice till golden brown.
2. Add chicken cubes and fry.
3. Add vegetables and fry.
4. Add pineapple cubes and remove from heat.
5. Mix together rest of the ingredients and bring it to boil and mix well.
6. Add this sauce to chicken and vegetables stir fry and cook together for one more minute.
7. Serve hot with plain rice.

Chicken ginger

Ingredients

Chicken 1 cup boneless cubes
Tomatoes 3 diced
Onion 1 sliced
Ginger ¼ cup matchsticks
Garlic cloves 6 sliced
Red chili powder ½ tea spoon
All spice powder or garam masala ½ tea spoon
Salt to taste
Oil ½ cup

Directions

1. Fry garlic slices and onion slices till golden brown.
2. Add chicken cubes and fry.
3. Add tomatoes and spices and fry.
4. Add finely cut ginger over chicken and serve hot.

Chicken with almond

Ingredients

Chicken 1 cup boneless cubes
Almond ½ cup blanched and split into two
Onion 1 diced
Green chilies ½ cup diced, remove seeds
Garlic cloves 10 sliced
Chicken broth 1 cup
Vinegar 2 table spoons
Corn flour ¼ cup
Soy sauce ½ cup gluten free
Salt and pepper to taste
Oil ¼ cup

Directions

1. Fry almonds and garlic till golden brown.
2. Add chicken and fry.
3. Add onion and green chilies and fry.
4. In a separate pan prepare sauce by mixing rest of the ingredients.
5. Mix chicken broth with corn flour, vinegar, salt, pepper, soy sauce and bring to boil and mix well.
6. Add it to the chicken and vegetables stir fries.
7. Serve hot with rice.

Chicken and broccoli with lemon sauce

Ingredients

Chicken 1 cup boneless cubes
Broccoli 1 cup cubes
Onion 1 diced
Garlic cloves 8 sliced
Lemon 4 table spoons
Chicken broth 1 cup
Corn flour ¼ cup
Soy sauce ¼ cup gluten free
Salt and pepper to taste

Directions

1. Fry garlic slices till golden brown.
2. Add chicken cubes and fry.
3. Add broccoli fry.
4. Add onion and fry.
5. In a separate pan prepare sauce.
6. Mix corn flour with broth, soy sauce, lemon juice, salt and pepper and bring to boil.
7. Add prepared sauce in chicken and vegetables stir fries and cook together for one more minute on high heat.
8. Serve hot with plain rice.

Chicken Manchurian

Ingredients

Chicken 2 cups boneless cubes
Garlic paste 2 table spoons
Green chili paste 1 table spoon
Tomato puree 1 cup
Chicken broth 1-2 cups
Vinegar 1 table spoon
Corn flour ½ cup
Soy sauce ½ cup gluten free
Salt and pepper to taste
Oil ¼ cup

Directions

1. Mix Chicken cubes with ginger paste, vinegar, green chili paste, soy sauce and corn flour and fry.
2. Add tomato puree, salt, pepper and broth and bring to boil.
3. Cover and simmer for five to ten minutes.
4. Serve hot with rice.

Chicken with orange

Ingredients

Chicken boneless cubes 1 cup
Orange 1 cup cubes
Onion 1 diced
Capsicum 1 diced
Chicken broth 1 cup
Garlic slices 8
Soy sauce ½ cup gluten free
Corn flour ¼ cup
Vinegar 3 table spoons
Salt and pepper to taste
Oil ¼ cup

Directions

1. Fry garlic slices till golden brown.
2. Add chicken cubes and fry.
3. Add capsicum and onion and fry.
4. Add orange cubes and move the pan away from stove.
5. Prepare sauce and mix corn flour with broth, vinegar, and soy sauce and bring to boil.
6. Add this prepared sauce to stir fried vegetables and chicken, mix well and cook for one more minute together on high heat.
7. Serve hot with rice.

Chicken with spinach

Ingredients

Chicken with bones 1 lb.
Spinach 3 cup chopped
Onion 2 sliced
Tomatoes 4 chopped
Ginger and garlic paste 3 table spoons
Red chili powder 1 tea spoon
Coriander seeds powder 1 tea spoon
Cumin seeds powder 1 tea spoon
Turmeric ½ tea spoon
Salt and pepper to taste
Oil ½ cup

Directions

1. Fry onion till golden brown.
2. Add tomatoes and ginger and garlic paste and fry till it gets mushy.
3. Add chicken and all the spices and fry.
4. Add 2 cups of water and bring to boil.
5. Simmer, cover and cook till chicken gets tender.
6. Add spinach and cook on high heat uncovered for few minutes.
7. Cover, simmer and cook on low heat for five to ten more minutes.

8. Serve hot with rice.

Chicken jalfrezy

Ingredients

Chicken 1 cup boneless cubes
Capsicum 1 cup diced
Cherry tomatoes 1 cup
Onion 1 cup diced
Green chili 1 chopped
Garlic cloves 10
Worcestershire sauce ½ cup
Mustard powder ½ teaspoon
Tomato puree 1 cup
Five spice mixor garam masala powder ½ tea spoon
Black pepper ½ tea spoon
Salt to taste
Oil ½ cup

Directions

1. Fry garlic slices till golden brown.
2. Add chicken and fry.
3. Add vegetables and fry.
4. Add rest of the ingredients and mix well.
5. Cook together for few minutes.
6. Serve hot with rice.

Baked chicken

Ingredients

Chicken cut in quarters 4
Yogurt ½ cup
Ginger and garlic paste 3 table spoons
Lemon juice 3 table spoons
Black pepper 1 tea spoon
Salt to taste
Almond powder ½ cup

Directions

1. Mix all the ingredients well and keep in the refrigerator for marinating.
2. Pre-heat oven at medium temperature and bake chicken till tender and acquires right color and texture.
3. Serve hot with salads and rice.

Chicken sash lick

Ingredients

Chicken 1 cup boneless cubes
Capsicum 1 cup diced
Tomatoes 1 cup diced
Onion 1 cup diced
Tomato sauce 3 tablespoons
Soy sauce ½ cup gluten free
Garlic paste 1 table spoon
Salt and pepper to taste
Olive oil 1 table spoon

Directions

1. Mix all the ingredients well and marinade for few hour in the refrigerator.
2. Thread these on skewers alternatingly and grill over charcoal till done.
3. Serve hot with rice.

Beef with saffron rice

Ingredients

Beef 1 lb. boneless cubes
Rice basmati long grains 3 cups wash and soak for half an hour
Onion 2 sliced
Tomatoes 4 chopped
Potatoes 2 cut in quarters and fry
Unsweetened yogurt 1 cup
Ginger and garlic paste 3 table spoons
Garam masala powder or five spice powder 1 tea spoon
Coriander seeds powder 1 tea spoon
Cumin seeds powder 1 tea spoon
Red chili powder 1 tea spoon
Star anise 2
Saffron few strands
Salt to taste
Oil 1 cup

Directions

1. Fry onion till golden brown in half of the given oil.
2. Add tomatoes and fry till mushy.
3. Add rest of the ingredients except rice, saffron, potatoes and remaining oil.

4. Add just enough water for the meat to get tender and bring to boil.
5. Cover, simmer and cook till meat gets tender.
6. Dry out any excess water remaining in the beef gravy and make it dry by cooking on high heat and stirring.
7. Drain out excess water from rice and cook it in a wide mouth pan.
8. Add four and a half cups of boiling water, remaining oil, saffron strands and salt to rice and bring it to a boil.
9. Cover and cook rice at medium heat till all the water dries.
10. Keep it over a pre-heated skillet for five to ten more minutes.
11. Take out half of the rice in some container and spread evenly the remaining half in the pan.
12. Pour the gravy layer over the rice layer and the taken out half rice layer over gravy layer. Top it with fried potatoes.
13. Keep over a warm skillet for further ten minutes.
14. Mix well and serve hot.

Chicken and chickpea curry

Ingredients

Chicken 1 lb. with bones
Chickpeas 1 cup boiled
Onion 1 sliced
Tomatoes 3 chopped
Garlic cloves 8 sliced
Red chili powder 1 tea spoon
Cumin seeds powder 1 tea spoon
Coriander seeds powder 1 tea spoon
Turmeric powder ½ tea spoon
Coriander leaves ½ chopped
Salt to taste
Oil ½ cup

Directions

1. Fry onion and garlic slices till golden brown.
2. Add tomatoes and fry till mushy.
3. Add chicken and fry.
4. Add chickpeas and spices and fry.
5. Add enough water for chicken to get tender and for required gravy.
6. Cover, simmer and cook till chicken gets tender.
7. Garnish with freshly chopped coriander leaves and serve hot with rice.

Chicken saffron rice

Ingredients

Onion paste ½ cup
Yogurt 1 cup
Chicken 1 cup boneless cubes
Rice 1 cup wash and soak for 30 minutes
Small cardamom 3
Mace powder ¼ tea spoon
Ginger and garlic paste 1 table spoon
Green chili paste 1 table spoon
Saffron few strands
Salt to taste
Oil ½ cup

Directions

1. Fry chicken, onion, ginger, garlic, green chili paste for few minutes.
2. Add yogurt, cardamom small, mace powder, saffron strands, rice, salt and two cups of boiling water and bring it to a boil.
3. Cover and cook over medium heat till all the water dries up.
4. Keep the pan over a pre heated skillet for ten more minutes.
5. Mix well and serve hot.

Chicken with garlic sauce

Ingredients

Chicken 1 cup boneless cubes
Capsicum 1 cup diced
Onion 1 cup diced
Carrots 1 cup diced
Garlic paste 2 table spoon
Vinegar ¼ cup
Chicken broth 2 cups
Corn flour ½ cup
Soy sauce ½ cup gluten free
Salt and pepper to taste
Oil ½ cup

Directions

1. Fry chicken in 1 tea spoon garlic paste and ¼ cup of oil.
2. Add onion, capsicum and carrots and fry.
3. Prepare a sauce and in a separate sauce pan fry remaining garlic paste.
4. Dissolve corn flour in chicken broth and add it to the garlic sauce pan.
5. Add vinegar, soy sauce, salt and pepper and bring it to a boil.
6. Add this sauce to chicken and serve hot with plain rice.

Spicy chicken with mixed vegetables

Ingredients

Chicken 1 lb. with bones
Onion 2 sliced
Tomatoes 4 chopped
Peas 1 cup
Potatoes 1 cup diced
Carrots 1 cup diced
Garlic 10 cloves sliced
Red chili powder 1 tea spoon
Cardamom small 5 whole Split open
Cinnamon stick 1 inch piece
Cumin seeds powder 1 tea spoon
Salt to taste
Oil ½ cup

Directions

1. Fry garlic slices and onion in oil till golden brown.
2. Add tomatoes and cook till mushy.
3. Add chicken, spices, salt and two cups water and bring to boil.
4. Mix well, cover, simmer and cook till chicken is half tender.
5. Add vegetables and cook till vegetables and chicken get tender.
6. Serve hot with rice.

Egg curry

Ingredients

Eggs 6 hard boiled and shelled
Yogurt 1 cup
Onion 2 fried golden brown
Tomatoes 2 chopped
Green chilies 2 chopped
Garlic cloves 8 sliced
Almond powder 2 table spoons
Cumin seeds powder 1 tea spoon
Coriander powder 1 tea spoon
Turmeric powder ½ tea spoon
Cinnamon powder ¼ tea spoon
Fresh coriander leaves ½ cup chopped
Salt to taste
Oil ½ cup

Directions

1. In two table spoon of oil fry whole garlic and green chilies.
2. Add chopped tomatoes and fry.
3. In a blender put this fried mixture, fried onion and yogurt and blend well.
4. Now in the same pan pour the remaining oil and fry this blended mixture.

5. Add all the spices and boiled eggs and fry.
6. Add enough water to make gravy of required consistency and bring it to a boil.
7. Mix well, cover, simmer and cook for ten more minutes.
8. Garnish with freshly chopped coriander leaves and serve hot with boiled rice.

Eggs and vegetables fried rice

Ingredients

Eggs 3
Rice 2 cups basmati long grains wash and soak for half an hour
Vegetables ½ cup each diced or julienne, carrots, onion, spring onion, cabbage, capsicum
Soy sauce ½ cup gluten free
Garlic cloves 8 sliced
Salt and pepper to taste
Oil ½ cup

Directions

1. Drain out excess water from rice.
2. Add three cups of boiling water, two tea spoons salt, ¼ cup soy sauce and ¼ cup oil in rice and cook covered at medium heat till all the water evaporates.
3. Keep rice over pre-heated skillet for five or ten more minutes.
4. Fry garlic slices in little oil till golden brown.
5. Add all the vegetables and remaining soy sauce and fry.
6. Add salt and pepper to taste and mix well and spread these fried vegetables over rice.
7. Fry eggs in little oil and keep mixing so that they are well cooked from all sides.

8. Add little salt and mix now spread cooked eggs over vegetable layer.
9. Mix rice, vegetables and eggs together and serve hot.

Scrambled spicy eggs

Ingredients

Eggs 6
Onion 3 sliced
Tomatoes 4 chopped
Green chilies 3 chopped
Red chili powder 1 tea spoon
Turmeric powder ½ tea spoon
Fresh coriander leaves 1 cup
Salt to taste
Oil ½ cup

Directions

1. Fry onion till lightly golden brown.
2. Add tomatoes and cook till mushy.
3. Add green chilies, turmeric powder, red chili powder, and salt and mix.
4. Add eggs and mix well and keep stirring so that eggs are cooked from all sides.
5. Add chopped coriander leaves and serve hot.

Beef with onion

Ingredients

Beef 1 cup boiled
Onion 1 cup diced
Garlic cloves 6 sliced
Lemon juice 2 table spoons
Oregano 1 table spoon
Salt and black pepper to taste
Oil ½ cup

Directions

1. Fry garlic slices till golden brown.
2. Add boiled beef and fry.
3. Add onion and fry.
4. Add lemon juice, oregano, salt and pepper and fry.
5. Serve hot with plain rice.

Chicken with chilies

Ingredients

Chicken 1 cup boneless cubes
Onion 1 diced
Garlic cloves 8 sliced
Chicken broth 1 cup
Green chilies ½ cup deseededcut length wise into two
Soy sauce ¼ cup gluten free
Corn flour ¼ cup
Salt and pepper to taste

Directions

1. Fry garlic slices in oil till golden brown.
2. Add chicken cubes and fry.
3. Add green chilies and onion and fry.
4. Add soy sauce, salt and pepper.
5. Mix corn flour in chicken broth and add this to chicken and bring it to a boil.
6. Cook for few more minutes and serve hot with plain rice.

Beef with chilies

Ingredients

Beef 1 cup boneless and boiled
Onion 1 cup diced
Green chilies ½ cup deseeded cut length wise into two
Soy sauce ½ cup gluten free
Beef broth 1 cup
Corn flour ¼ cup
Soy sauce ½ cup
Garlic cloves 6 sliced
Salt and pepper to taste
Vinegar 2 table spoons
Oil ½ cup

Directions

1. Fry garlic slices till golden brown.
2. Add boiled beef and fry.
3. Add onion and green chilies and fry.
4. Add soy sauce, salt, pepper and vinegar and fry.
5. Mix corn flour in beef broth and add this to the cooking pan and stir well.
6. Bring it to a boil and cook for few more minutes and serve hot.

Chicken and potato cutlets

Ingredients

Chicken 1 cup boiled cubes
Potatoes 3 boiled and mashed
Green chilies 3 chopped
Egg 1 well beaten
Coriander leaves 1 cup chopped
Lemon juice 2 table spoons
Cumin seeds 1 table spoon roasted over a skillet
Salt and pepper to taste
Oil for shallow frying

Directions

1. Mix all the ingredients well except oil and egg.
2. Make disc of the mixture with the help of your palms and flatten it to make it half inch thick.
3. Dip in beaten egg and shallow fry from both sides till golden brown.
4. Serve hot.

Chicken BBQ

Ingredients

Chicken 2 lbs. boneless 1 inch cubes
Cream ½ cup
Ginger and garlic paste ¼ cup
Yogurt ½ cup
Green chili paste 2 table spoons
Raw papaya paste 1 table spoon
Red chili powder 1 tea spoon
Cumin seeds powder 1 tea spoon
Coriander seeds powder 1 tea spoon
All spice mix or garam masala powder 1 tea spoon
Salt to taste

Directions

1. Mix all the ingredients well and marinade for few hour preferably one day in the refrigerator.
2. Thread chicken pieces on skewers and grill over charcoal till done.
3. Serve hot.

Beef BBQ

Ingredients

Beef 2 lb. boneless 1 inch cubes
Yogurt ½ cup
Vinegar ½ cup
Ginger and garlic paste ¼ cup
Meat tenderizer 1 table spoon or raw papaya paste 1 table spoon
Onion paste 1 table spoon
Green chili paste 2 table spoons
Coriander leaves paste 3 table spoons
Cardamom small powder 1 tea spoon
Mace powder ½ tea spoon
Salt to taste
Olive oil 3 table spoons

Directions

1. Mix all the ingredients well together and keep for marinating in refrigerator for few hours but preferably for one day.
2. Thread beef pieces over skewers and grill over charcoal till done.
3. Serve hot.

Chicken BBQ kebabs

Ingredients

Chicken 2 lb. boneless chunks
Onion 3
Green chilies 5
Ginger 2 inch piece
Garlic cloves 12
Coriander leaves 1 cup
Coriander seeds 1 table spoon roasted over skillet
Cumin seeds 1 table spoon roasted over skillet
Mustard powder 1 tea spoon
Five spice powder or garam masala powder or any spice of choice 1 tea spoon
Yogurt 3 table spoons
Lemon juice 3 table spoons
Salt and pepper to taste
Olive oil 1 table spoon

Directions

1. Chop all the ingredients well together in a chopper.
2. Spread the chopped mixture with the help of your palms over skewers.
3. Grill over charcoal grill till done.
4. Serve hot.

Beef BBQ kebabs

Ingredients

Beef 2 lb. boneless
Onion 4
Yogurt ¼ cup
Green chilies 5
Coriander leaves 1 cup
Ginger 2 inch piece
Garlic 12 cloves
Coriander seeds 1 table spoon
Cumin seeds 1 table spoon
Five spice mix or garam masala mix or any spice of choice 1 tea spoon
Cream ¼ cup
Corn meal ½ cup
Salt to taste

Directions

1. Chop all the ingredients well in a chopper.
2. Spread the chopped mixture nicely over skewers with the help of your palm.
3. Grill over charcoal grill till done.
4. Serve hot.

Beef steak

Ingredients

Beef undercut individual pieces 4 pieces
Ginger and garlic paste 1 table spoons
Molasses 1 table spoon
Lemon juice 2 table spoons
Coconut cream powder 1 table spoon
Salt and pepper to taste
Olive oil 3 table spoons

Directions

1. Marinade beef pieces in all the ingredients listed and keep in the refrigerator for 24 hours.
2. On a grill pan spread out the marinated beef pieces and cover and grill one side till done.
3. Turn it over and cook other half till done.
4. Serve hot with grilled vegetables and mashed potatoes.

Chicken steak

Ingredients

Chicken 4 steak pieces
Ginger paste 1 table spoon
Green chili paste 1 table spoon
Lemon juice 2 table spoon
Red chili powder 1 tea spoon
Cumin seeds powder 1 tea spoon
Honey 1 table spoon
Yogurt 4 table spoons
Tomato sauce 1 table spoon
Salt and pepper to taste
Butter melted 3 table spoons

Directions

1. Marinade chicken pieces for at least 24 hour in all the listed ingredients and keep it cold in the refrigerator.
2. Spread chicken pieces over grill pan evenly and grill on both sides evenly and keep covered while cooking to reduce moisture loss during cooking.
3. Serve hot with grilled vegetables and mashed potatoes.

Beef and gram pulses curry

Ingredients

Beef 1 lb. boneless pieces
Gram pulses 1 cup wash and soak for one hour
Onion 2 sliced
Tomatoes 4 chopped
Ginger and garlic paste 2 table spoons
Cinnamon stick 1 inch piece
Cloves 4
Cardamom small 4
Cumin seeds powder 1 table spoon
Red chili powder 1 tea spoon
Salt and pepper to taste
Coriander leaves ½ cup chopped
Oil ½ cup

Directions

1. Fry onion slices and whole spices in oil till golden brown.
2. Add ginger and garlic paste and tomatoes and fry till mushy.
3. Add all the remaining ingredients and fry.
4. Add enough water for meat and gram pulses to get tender.
5. Mix well, cover, simmer and cook till meat and gram pulses get tender.

6. Garnish with freshly chopped coriander leaves and serve hot with rice or corn bread.

Chicken with tomatoes

Ingredients

Chicken 1 lb. boneless pieces
Tomatoes 6 chopped
Green chilies 8 chopped deseed if you want less hot
Ginger and garlic paste 2 table spoons
Coriander leaves 1 cup chopped
Turmeric powder ½ tea spoon
Salt to taste
Five spice powder or garam masala powder 1 tea spoon
Oil ½ cup

Directions

1. Fry chicken with ginger and garlic paste.
2. Add tomatoes and fry till tomatoes are mushy.
3. Add 1 cup water bring to boil, cover and simmer.
4. When half tender, add green chilies, cover and cook till tender.
5. Add chopped coriander leaves and fry for few minutes.
6. Serve hot with rice.

Minced beef with capsicum

Ingredients

Beef minced 1 lb.
Capsicum 2 diced
Onion 2 sliced
Tomatoes 4 chopped
Ginger and garlic paste 3 table spoons
Cumin seeds powder 1 table spoon
Turmeric powder ½ tea spoon
Coriander powder 1 tea spoon
Red chili powder 1 tea spoon
Cardamom small 6
Salt to taste
Oil ½ cup

Directions

1. Fry onion and cardamom small till golden brown.
2. Add tomatoes and ginger and garlic paste and cook till mushy.
3. Add minced meat and all the spices and fry.
4. Add capsicum and fry.
5. Serve hot.

Chicken with capsicum

Ingredients

Chicken 1 lb. boneless pieces
Tomatoes 4 chopped
Onion 2 sliced
Ginger and garlic paste 2 table spoons
Cumin seeds powder 1 table spoon
Capsicum 2 diced
Red chili powder 1 tea spoon
Salt to taste
Oil ½ cup

Directions

1. Fry onion slices till golden brown.
2. Add tomatoes, ginger and garlic paste, chicken, cumin seeds powder, red chili powder and salt and fry.
3. Add one cup of water and bring to boil.
4. Mix well, cover, simmer and cook till tender.
5. Add diced capsicum and fry, simmer and let it cook for few more minutes.
6. Serve hot.

Mined beef with potatoes

Ingredients

Beef minced 1 lb.
Potatoes 3 diced
Onion 2 sliced
Tomatoes 4 chopped
Cardamom small 5
Ginger and garlic paste 3 table spoons
Green chili paste 2 table spoons
Cloves 4
Cinnamon stick 1 inch piece
Cumin seeds powder 1 table spoon
Turmeric powder ½ tea spoon
Yogurt ½ cup
Coriander leaves ½ cup chopped
Salt to taste
Oil ½ cup

Directions

1. Fry onion and cardamom till onion turns golden brown.
2. Add tomatoes, green chili paste, ginger and garlic paste, salt and fry till tomatoes are mushy.
3. Add minced meat, yogurt, salt and all the spices and fry.

4. Add potatoes and one cup of water and bring to boil.
5. Mix well, cover, simmer and cook till potatoes get tender.
6. Garnish coriander leaves and serve hot.

Mutton and potato curry

Ingredients

Mutton 1 lb. leg pieces
Potatoes 3 cut in quarters
Onion 2 sliced and fried till golden brown
Tomatoes 2 chopped
Yogurt 1 cup
Small cardamoms 6 split them open
Cloves 5
Cinnamon stick 1 inch piece
Ginger and garlic paste 3 table spoons
Red chili powder 1 tea spoon
Cumin seed powder 1 table spoon
Turmeric powder ½ tea spoon
Salt to taste
Fresh coriander leaves ½ cup chopped
Oil ½ cup

Directions

1. Fry mutton with ginger and garlic paste and whole spices.
2. Add tomatoes and fry till tomatoes get mushy.
3. Add rest of the spices and enough water for meat to get tender.
4. Mix well, cover, simmer, and cook till meat is almost done.

5. Blend yogurt with fried onions and 1 cup water.
6. Add blended mixture and potatoes and salt to the mutton pan and cook till potatoes get tender.
7. Garnish with freshly chopped coriander leaves and serve hot with rice.

Minced beef and spinach

Ingredients

Beef minced 1 lb.
Spinach 3 cups
Onion 2 sliced
Tomatoes 4 chopped
Ginger and garlic paste 3 table spoons
Yogurt ½ cup
Whole spices of choice, cardamom small, cloves, cinnamon stick, 1 table spoon
Red chili powder 1 tea spoon
Cumin seeds powder 1 table spoon
Salt to taste
Oil ½ cup

Directions

1. Fry onion slices with whole spices till onion turns golden brown.
2. Add tomatoes, ginger and garlic paste and fry till mushy.
3. Add minced beef, yogurt and rest of the ingredients and keep frying for few more minutes.
4. Add 1 cup water and bring to boil.
5. Mix well, cover, simmer and cook for ten to fifteen more minutes.
6. Serve hot with rice.

Minced beef with peas

Ingredients

Beef minced 1 lb.
Peas 1 cups
Onion 2 sliced
Tomatoes 4 chopped
Ginger and garlic paste 2 table spoons
Yogurt ½ cup
Whole spices of choice 1 table spoon
Cumin seeds powder 1 table spoon
Red chili powder 1 tea spoon
Salt to taste
Oil ½ cup

Directions

1. Fry onion and whole spices till onion turns golden brown.
2. Add tomatoes and ginger and garlic paste till tomatoes get mushy.
3. Add yogurt, minced meat, peas and rest of the ingredients and 1 cup water and mix well and bring to boil.
4. Cover, simmer and cook for fifteen minutes.
5. Uncover and fry for few more minutes.
6. Serve hot.

Chicken, peas and potato rice

Ingredients

Chicken 1 cup boneless cubes
Peas 1 cup
Potatoes 1 cup diced
Onion 1 sliced
Tomatoes 3 chopped
Red chili powder 1 tea spoon
Cumin seeds powder 1 tea spoon
Garlic clove 6 sliced
Salt to taste
Oil ½ cup

Directions

1. Fry onion and garlic in oil till they become golden brown.
2. Add tomatoes and fry till mushy.
3. Add chicken and fry.
4. Add peas, potatoes, spices and 1 cup water and bring to boil.
5. Mix well, cover, simmer and cook on low heat till potatoes get tender.
6. Serve hot with rice.

Chicken salad

Ingredients

Chicken boneless cubes 1 cup
Carrots 1 cup boiled
Potatoes 1 cup boiled
Peas 1 cup boiled
Cream cheese ½ cup
Coconut cream ½ cup
Honey 2 table spoon
Salt and pepper to taste
Sesame seeds oil 3 table spoons

Directions

1. Fry chicken in little oil till golden brown.
2. Mix all the ingredients well in a mixing bowl and serve cold.

Beef salad

Ingredients

Beef 1 cup boneless small cubes boiled and fried
Corn 1 cup
Potatoes 1 cup boiled
Chickpeas 1 cup boiled
Red beans 1 cup boiled
Mustard sauce 1 table spoon roasted over skillet
Olive oil 3 table spoons
Lemon juice 2 table spoons
Salt and pepper to taste

Directions

1. Mix all the ingredients well and serve cold.

Chicken and vegetables soup

Ingredients

Chicken 1 cup boneless cubes
Quinoa 1 cup boiled
Mixed vegetables 1 cup
Garlic 6 cloves
Tomatoes 3
Onion 1
Salt and pepper to taste
Olive oil 3 table spoon

Directions

1. Mix all the ingredients and cook in enough water to make soup.
2. Blend all the ingredients well in a blender.
3. Bring it to a boil and add more water if needed.
4. Cook for ten more minutes and serve hot with gluten free croutons.

Beef with mixed vegetables soup

Ingredients

Beef 1 cup cubes
Mixed lentils ½ cup
Tomatoes 4
Potato 1
Onion 1
Coriander leaves 1 cup
Olives ½ cup
Salt and pepper to taste

Directions

1. Mix all the ingredients and cook in enough water till tender.
2. Blend all the ingredients well in a blender.
3. Bring it to a boil and add more water if needed.
4. Cook for ten more minutes and serve hot.

Chicken with baby corns

Ingredients

Chicken 1 cup boneless cubes
Baby corn 1 cup
Cherry tomatoes 1 cup
Baby onion 1 cup
Lemon juice 2 table spoons
Mustard powder ½ tea spoon
Garlic 6 cloves sliced
Worcestershire sauce ½ cup
Salt and pepper to taste
Oil ½ cup

Directions

1. Fry garlic slices till golden brown.
2. Add chicken cubes and fry.
3. Add onion and baby corn and fry.
4. Add cherry tomatoes and fry.
5. Add rest of the ingredients, cover and fry for five more minutes.
6. Serve hot.

Chicken with mushrooms

Ingredients

Chicken 1 cup boneless cubes
Mushrooms 1 cup sliced
Almond milk 1 cup
Garlic cloves 6 sliced
Lemon juice 2 table spoons
Salt and pepper to taste

Directions

1. Fry garlic slices till golden brown.
2. Add chicken and fry.
3. Add mushrooms and fry.
4. Add rest of the ingredients and cook covered for five more minutes.
5. Serve hot.

Beef with lentils

Ingredients

Beef 1 cup boneless cubes
Mixed lentils 1 cup
Onion 1 sliced
Tomatoes 3 chopped
Ginger and garlic paste 2 table spoons
Herbs and spices of choice 1 table spoon
Salt and pepper to taste
Oil ½ cup

Directions

1. Fry garlic and onion till golden brown.
2. Add tomatoes and ginger and garlic paste and fry till mushy.
3. Add rest of the ingredients and 3 cups of water and cook till tender.
4. Serve hot with rice.

Creamy chicken pasta

Ingredients

Chicken 1 cup boneless cubes
Gluten free pasta 3 cups boiled and strained
Avocado 1 peeled and sliced
Onion 1 diced
Garlic cloves 8 sliced
Cream cheese 1 cup
Tomato puree 1 cup
Basil 1 table spoon
Worcestershire sauce 3 table spoons
Salt and pepper to taste
Oil ½ cup

Directions

1. Fry garlic in oil till golden brown.
2. Add chicken cubes and fry.
3. Add Worcestershire sauce and fry.
4. Add diced onion and fry.
5. Add avocado slices and fry.
6. Add rest of the ingredients.
7. Mix well, cover, simmer and cook for five more minutes.
8. Serve hot.

Baked beef pasta

Ingredients

Beef 1 cup boneless cubes boiled
Onion 1 cup diced
Mushrooms 1 cup sliced
Parsley 1 table spoon
Garlic cloves 6 sliced
Corn meal ½ cup
Gluten free pasta of choice 3 cups boiled and strained
Milk 1-2 cups
Lemon juice 3 table spoons
Salt and pepper to taste
Olive oil ½ cup

Directions

1. Fry garlic in half oil till golden brown
2. Add boiled beef and fry.
3. Add onions and mushrooms and fry.
4. In a separate sauce pan fry corn meal in remaining oil for few minutes.
5. Add milk slowly stirring continuously so that lumps are not formed.
6. Add salt, pepper and parsley and mix well.
7. Add this sauce to beef stir fry and add all the remaining ingredients.
8. Mix well, cover, simmer and cook together for five more minutes.

9. Serve hot.

Sweet and sour spaghetti

Ingredients

Beef minced 1 cup
Capsicum 1 cup chopped
Garlic cloves 8 sliced
Onion 1 cup chopped
Tomatoes 1 cup chopped
Lemon juice 4 table spoons
Honey 4 table spoons
Cilantro 1 table spoon
Gluten free spaghetti 3 cups boiled and strained
Beef broth 1 cup
Salt and pepper to taste
Olive oil ½ cup

Directions

1. Fry garlic slices in oil till golden brown.
2. Add onion and fry.
3. Add tomatoes and fry till mushy.
4. Add minced meat and fry.
5. Add rest of the ingredients.
6. Mix well, cover, simmer and cook together for five more minutes.
7. Serve hot.

Gluten-free tortillas

Ingredients

Rice powder 2 cups
Corn meal 2 cups
Corn flour 1 cup
Egg 2
Cumin seeds powder 1 table spoon
Cilantro 1 table spoon
Salt and pepper to taste
Oil ½ cup

Directions

1. Except oil mix all the ingredients well together and knead (use milk if needed).
2. Using rolling pin and board roll it using little dry corn meal for easy rolling.
3. Cook it over pre-heated skillet and spread oil on each side with the help of a spoon.
4. Serve hot.

Potato tortillas

Ingredients

Potatoes 5 boiled and mashed
Corn flour 2 cups
Coriander leaves fresh 1 cup chopped
Red chili powder 1 tea spoon
Mustard seeds 1 table spoon
Salt and pepper to taste
Oil ½ cup

Directions

1. Mix all the ingredients well and knead (if required add some milk).
2. Using rolling pin and board roll it to make a tortilla using little extra corn flour if needed.
3. Cook it over a pre heated skillet and turn over to make sure it is cooked from all sides.
4. Spread oil on both sides while cooking.
5. Serve hot.

Corn and egg tortillas

Ingredients

Corn meal 4 cups
Eggs 2
Green chilies 2 chopped
Garlic paste 1 table spoon
Salt and pepper to taste
Oil ½ cup

Directions

1. Mix all the ingredients together and knead (use milk or extra corn meal if needed).
2. Roll it using a rolling pin and board.
3. Cook it over a pre-heated skillet turning over and cooking from all sides.
4. Spread oil on both sides.
5. Serve hot.

Creamy tomato and egg soup

Ingredients

Tomatoes 8 chopped
Onion 2 chopped
Coriander leaves 1 cup chopped
Egg 1 well beaten
Garlic 5 cloves
Vinegar 2 table spoons
Molasses 2 table spoons
Fresh cream ½ cup
Salt and pepper to taste
Olive oil ½ cup

Directions

1. In oil fry all the vegetables.
2. Add enough water and all the ingredients except egg and cream and cook till tender.
3. Blend all together.
4. Bring to boil and add more water if needed.
5. Add well beaten and stir quickly.
6. Add cream and mix.
7. Serve hot.

Chicken and mushroom soup

Ingredients

Chicken 1cup boneless chopped
Mushrooms 2 cups sliced
Onion 1 chopped
Garlic cloves 6 chopped
Corn flour 1 cup
Chicken broth 4-6 cups
Soy sauce ½ cup gluten free
Vinegar 3 table spoons
Salt and pepper to taste
Sesame seeds oil 4 table spoons

Directions

1. Fry garlic in oil and add chopped chicken and fry.
2. Add mushrooms and onion and fry.
3. Dissolve corn flour in broth and add rest of the ingredients and bring to boil and cook together for few minutes.
4. Serve hot.

Corn and chicken rice

Ingredients

Chicken 1 cup boneless cubes
Corn 1 cup
Rice 2 cups basmati long grain, wash and soak in water
Garlic cloves 7 sliced
Onion 1 chopped
Tomatoes 3 chopped
Green chili paste 1 table spoon
Salt and pepper to taste
Oil ½ cup

Directions

1. Fry garlic in oil till golden brown.
2. Add onion and fry.
3. Add chicken and fry.
4. Add corn and fry.
5. Add rest of the ingredients and 3 cups of boiling water.
6. Mix well, cover, simmer and cook till rice get dry.
7. Keep the pan over pre-heated skillet for five to ten more minutes.
8. Serve hot.

Fried chicken

Ingredients

Chicken 1lb. with bones and skin
Rice flour ½ cup
Corn flour ½ cup
Gram flour ½ cup
Ginger and garlic paste 2 table spoons
Vinegar 3 table spoons
Cumin seeds powder 1 table spoon
Green chili paste 1 table spoon
Salt and pepper to taste
Oil for deep frying

Directions

1. Mix salt, pepper, rice flour, corn flour and gram flour and keep aside for chicken coating.
2. Marinade chicken in rest of the ingredients except oil for few hours.
3. Press each chicken piece on dry coating and coat it properly from all sides.
4. Fry each piece till golden brown.
5. Serve hot.

Chicken and tomato curry

Ingredients

Chicken 1 lb. small pieces with bones
Tomatoes 6 grill over grill pan
Green chilies 4 grill over grill pan
Curry leaves few if available
Garlic 8 cloves grill over grill pan
Onion 1 grill over grill pan
Sesame seeds 3 table spoons roasted over skillet
Yogurt ½ cup
Red chili powder 1 tea spoon
Coriander seeds powder 1 tea spoon
Cumin seeds powder 1 tea spoon
Coriander leaves ½ cup chopped
Salt to taste
Oil ½ cup

Directions

1. Blend all the grilled and roasted ingredients well in a blender.
2. Marinade chicken in yogurt, red chili powder, cumin seeds powder, coriander seeds powder for some time.
3. Fry chicken and add blended mixture.
4. Mix well, cover, simmer and add enough water to make gravy.

5. Cook till chicken gets tender.
6. Garnish with freshly chopped coriander leaves and serve hot with rice.

Chicken green curry

Ingredients

Chicken 1 lb. small pieces with bones
Coconut powder 3 table spoons
Garlic cloves 8
Green chilies 6
Coriander leaves 1 cup
Cumin seeds powder 1 table spoon
Salt and pepper to taste
Pea nuts ¼ cup roasted peanut powder
Oil ½ cup

Directions

1. Blend together green chilies, coriander leaves, garlic, cumin seeds, coconut powder in little water.
2. Fry this blended mixture with chicken.
3. Add rest of the ingredients and fry.
4. Add enough water to make gravy.
5. Mix well, cover, simmer and cook till chicken gets tender.
6. Serve hot with rice.

Chicken coconut curry

Ingredients

Chicken boneless cubes 1 cup
Coconut milk 1 cup
Tomato puree 1 cup
Ginger and garlic paste 1 table spoon
Green chili paste 1 table spoon
Cumin seeds powder 1 table spoon
Coriander leaves ½ cup chopped
Salt to taste
Oil ½ cup

Direction

1. Fry chicken with ginger and garlic paste and green chili paste
2. Add rest of the ingredients and fry.
3. Add enough water to make gravy.
4. Mix well, cover, simmer and cook till tender.
5. Garnish with freshly chopped coriander leaves and serve hot with rice.

Grilled chicken with vegetables

Ingredients

Chicken 4 boneless large chunks
Vegetables mixed 1 cup of choice, add 1 table spoon vinegar and little salt and pepper
Honey 2 table spoons
Ginger paste 2 table spoons
Yogurt ¼ cup
Lemon juice 2 table spoon
Almond powder 2 table spoon
Salt and pepper to taste
Oil 4 table spoon

Directions

1. Except vegetables mix all the ingredients well and keep in the refrigerator for marinating for some time.
2. Grill these chicken pieces over a grill pan on both sides.
3. Grill the vegetables and serve hot together.

Roast chicken with stir fried vegetables

Ingredients

Chicken quarters 4
Mixed vegetables of choice 2-4 cups
Yogurt ½ cup
Lemon juice 4 table spoons
Green chili paste 2 table spoons
Molasses 1 table spoon
Ginger and garlic paste 2 table spoons
Mustard powder 1 tea spoon
White pepper 1 tea spoon
Salt to taste
Oil 3 table spoons

Directions

1. Mix all the ingredients together except vegetables and oil.
2. Keep chicken in the refrigerator for marinating.
3. Roast chicken in the pre-heated oven till done.
4. Stir fry vegetables in oil and little salt and pepper.
5. Serve hot.

Minced meat and potato cutlet

Ingredients

Minced meat 1 cup
Potatoes 4 boiled and mashed
Onion 1 chopped
Green chilies 3 chopped
Coriander leaves 1 cup chopped
Egg 1 well beaten
Salt and pepper to taste
Oil for shallow frying

Directions

1. Fry onion in little oil till soft.
2. Add minced meat and fry.
3. Add green chilies and fry
4. Add this fried minced meat to mashed potatoes and mix.
5. Add coriander leaves, salt and pepper and mix well.
6. Take a handful and make a round cutlet of the mixture.
7. Dip it in well beaten egg and shallow fry from both sides till golden brown in a pre-heated fry pan of oil.
8. Serve hot.

Spicy prawn rice

Ingredients

Prawn 1 cup de veined
Rice 2 cups, wash and soak for 30 minutes
Green chili paste 1 table spoon
Tomato puree ½ cup
Coconut milk ½ cup
Ginger and garlic paste 1 table spoon
Red chili powder 1 tea spoon
Coriander leaves ½ cup chopped
Cumin seeds powder 1 tea spoon
Salt to taste
Oil ½ cup

Directions

1. Fry prawns in ginger and garlic paste and green chili paste till done.
2. Add rest of the ingredients and three cups of boiling water.
3. Mix well, cover, simmer and cook till done.
4. Keep the pan over pre heated skillet for five to ten minutes.
5. Serve hot.

Sweet and sour prawns

Ingredients

Prawns 1 cup
Egg 1 well beaten
Corn flour ¾ cup
Soy sauce ½ cup gluten free
Tomato sauce ½ cup
Honey 4 table spoon
Vinegar 3 table spoon
Mixed vegetables 1 cup diced, onion, carrots, capsicum
Garlic paste 1 table spoon
Salt and pepper to taste
Oil ½ cup

Directions

1. Add ½ cup corn flour, garlic paste, little salt, little pepper, 2 table spoons soy sauce in well beaten egg and mix well.
2. Marinade prawns in egg mixture for some time.
3. Deep fry prawns till done.
4. Fry vegetables in oil and add fried prawns.
5. Make a sauce by mixing rest of the ingredients and little water and bring it to a boil.
6. Add this prepared sauce to vegetables and prawns and mix well and serve hot with rice.

Chicken spicy BBQ

Ingredients

Chicken quarters 4
Yogurt ¼ cup
Lemon juice 4 table spoons
Green chili paste 2 table spoons
Ginger and garlic paste 2 table spoons
Cumin seeds powder 1 table spoon
Coriander seeds powder 1 tea spoon
Mace powder ¼ tea spoon
Salt and pepper to taste
Sesame seeds oil 2 table spoons

Directions

1. Mix all the ingredients well and marinade chicken in the mix for few hours.
2. Use skewers to fasten chicken pieces and grill over charcoal from all sides till done.
3. Serve hot.

Mutton BBQ chops

Ingredients

Mutton chops 1 lb.
Five spice mix 1 tea spoon
Vinegar ¼ cup
Ginger and garlic paste 3 table spoons
Yogurt ¼ cup
Raw papaya paste or meat tenderizer 1 table spoon
Salt to taste

Directions

1. Marinade mutton in the listed ingredients for some time.
2. Thread mutton chops over skewers and grill over charcoal till done.
3. Serve hot.

Chicken gluten-free pizza

Ingredients

Corn meal ½ cup
Rice flour ½ cup
Potato flour ½ cup
Yeast 1 table spoon
Egg 1
Milk ¼ cup warm
Butter 1 table spoon
Sugar 1 tea spoon
Salt to taste
Fried chicken chunks 1 cup
Mixed vegetables 1 cup
Cheese shredded 1 cup
Pizza sauce ½ cup

Directions

1. Except last four listed ingredients knead all the ingredients together well and keep it covered at a warm place for some time to rise.
2. Pre heat oven at medium heat.
3. Spread the kneaded mixture with the help of your hands over a pizza baking tray.
4. Spread pizza sauce over it.
5. Spread selected diced vegetables over it.
6. Spread chicken chunks over it.

7. Spread shredded cheese over it.
8. Bake it for 10-15 minutes or till done.
9. Serve hot.

Mutton grilled chops

Ingredients

Mutton chops 1 lb.
Onion paste 1 table spoon
Green chili paste 1 table spoon
Ginger and garlic paste 2 table spoons
Yogurt ¼ cup
Lemon juice 2 table spoons
Raw papaya paste 1 table spoon
Red chili powder 1 tea spoon
Cumin seeds powder 1 table spoon
Salt and pepper to taste
Oil 2 table spoons

Directions

1. Marinade mutton in the listed ingredients for few hours.
2. Grill these over grill pan on both sides till done.
3. Serve hot.

Mutton roast

Ingredients

Mutton leg small 1
Ginger and garlic paste 3 table spoons
Yogurt ½ cup
Vinegar ½ cup
Five spice powder or garam masala powder 1 tea spoon
Raw papaya paste 2 table spoons
Green chili paste 2 table spoons
Salt to taste
Oil 2 table spoons

Directions

1. Marinade mutton leg in all the listed ingredients for 24 hours.
2. Roast it in a pre-heated oven till done.
3. Serve hot.

Mutton and potato curry

Ingredients

Mutton 1 lb. leg pieces small
Onion 2 sliced
Tomatoes 4 chopped
Ginger and garlic paste 3 table spoons
Potatoes 2 cut in quarters
Red chili powder 1 tea spoon
Coriander seeds powder 1 tea spoon
Five spice powder or garam masala powder 1 tea spoon
Salt to taste
Oil ½ cup

Directions

1. Fry onion in oil till golden brown.
2. Add tomatoes and ginger and garlic paste and fry till mushy.
3. Add rest of the ingredients except potatoes and fry for five minutes.
4. Add enough water for mutton to get tender, cover, simmer and cook till half tender.
5. When half cooked, add potatoes, cover, simmer and cook till tender.
6. Add extra water to make gravy and bring it to a boil.
7. Simmer and cook for ten more minutes.
8. Serve hot with rice.

Mutton and okra curry

Ingredients

Mutton leg 1 lb. small pieces
Okra ½ lb. fried in little oil
Onion 2 sliced
Tomatoes 4 chopped
Ginger and garlic paste 2 table spoons
Red chili powder 1 tea spoon
Cumin seeds powder 1 tea spoon
Coriander powder 1 tea spoon
Five spice powder or garam masala powder ½ tea spoon
Coriander leaves ½ cup chopped
Salt to taste
Oil ½ cup

Directions

1. Fry onion till golden brown.
2. Add chopped tomatoes and ginger and garlic paste and fry till mushy.
3. Add mutton and rest of the ingredients except okra and fry.
4. Add enough water for meat to get tender, mix well, cover, simmer and cook till tender.
5. Add fried okra and mix.
6. Add chopped coriander and serve hot with rice.

Mutton with mixed vegetables

Ingredients

Mutton leg 1 lb. small pieces
Onion 1 sliced
Ginger and garlic paste 2 table spoons
Yogurt ½ cup
Tomatoes 2 chopped
Salt to taste
Herbs and spices according to choice
Vegetables mixed 2 cups of choice
Oil ½ cup

Directions

1. Fry onion till golden brown.
2. Add mutton and yogurt and fry.
3. Add rest of the ingredients except vegetables and fry.
4. Add enough water for meat to get tender and cook on low heat till meat gets tender.
5. Add vegetables and cook for ten more minutes.
6. Serve hot.

Mutton spicy rice

Ingredients

Mutton leg 1 lb. small pieces
Yogurt 1 cup
Onion 1 sliced
Green chili paste 2 table spoons
Tomatoes 3 chopped
Ginger and garlic paste 2 table spoons
Whole spices 1 table spoon, small cardamom, large cardamom, cloves, cinnamon, bay leaf, star anise
Rice 3 cups long grains basmati wash and soak for 30 minutes
Salt to taste
Oil ½ cup

Directions

1. Fry onion and whole spices in oil till onion turns golden brown in color.
2. Add tomatoes, ginger and garlic paste and green chili paste and fry.
3. Add mutton and yogurt and fry.
4. Add enough water for meat to get tender and cook on low heat.
5. Add rest of the ingredients, four and a half cups of boiling water and mix well, cover and cook on medium heat till dry.

6. Keep it over a pre heated skillet for five to ten more minutes.
7. Serve hot.

Minced meat Pizza

Ingredients

Beef minced 1 cup
Onion 1 chopped
Garlic paste 1 table spoon
Mixed vegetables of choice 1 cup
Pizza sauce ½ cup
Cheese 1 cup shredded
Salt and pepper to taste
Corn flour ½ cup
Rice flour ½ cup
Tapioca flour ½ cup
Yeast 1 table spoon
Sugar 1 tea spoon
Egg 1 well beaten
Butter 1 table spoon
Milk 1/4 cup warm

Directions

1. Mix eight last listed ingredients together and keep in a warm place to rise.
2. Fry onion in oil till tender.
3. Add Minced beef, garlic paste, salt and pepper and mix well and fry.
4. Spread pizza dough over a pizza tray evenly.
5. Spread pizza sauce over it.

6. Add minced meat and cheese.
7. Add mixed vegetables and bake in a pre-heated oven for 10-15 minutes or till done.
8. Serve hot.

Mutton BBQ

Ingredients

Mutton 1 lb. leg pieces small
Ginger and garlic paste 2 table spoons
Onion paste 2 table spoons
Green chili paste 2 table spoons
Cumin seeds powder 1 table spoon
Yogurt ¼ cup
Raw papaya paste or meat tenderizer 1 table spoon
Vinegar 3 table spoons
Salt and pepper to taste

Directions

1. Thread mutton pieces over skewers and grill over charcoal till done.
2. Serve hot.

Mutton green coconut curry

Ingredients

Mutton leg 1 lb. small pieces
Coconut milk 1 cup
Green chilies 5
Coriander leaves 1 cup
Cumin seeds 1 table spoon
Onion 1
Garlic cloves 12
Salt and pepper to taste
Yogurt 1 cup
Oil ½ cup

Directions

1. Blend green chilies, onion, coriander leaves, garlic, and cumin seeds in a little water.
2. Fry mutton in oil and blended mixture for few minutes.
3. Add rest of the ingredients and mix well.
4. Add enough water to make gravy and to make meat tender.
5. Cover, simmer and cook till tender.
6. Serve hot with rice.

Mutton jalfrezy

Ingredients

Mutton leg 1 lb. small pieces
Tomato puree 1 cup
Capsicum 1 cup diced
Cherry tomatoes 1 cup whole
Onion 1 cup diced
Worcestershire sauce ½ cup
Mustard powder ½ tea spoon
Five spice powder or garam masala powder ½ tea spoon
Cumin seeds powder ½ tea spoon
Coriander seeds powder ½ tea spoon
Garlic cloves 12 sliced
Salt and black pepper to taste
Oil ½ cup

Directions

1. Fry garlic slices till golden brown in half oil.
2. Add mutton and fry.
3. Add rest of the ingredients except vegetables.
4. Add enough water for meat to get tender.
5. Mix well, cover, simmer and cook on low heat till meat gets tender.
6. Fry vegetables in a separate fryer in remaining oil.

7. Add these to mutton, mix well and cook together for few more minutes.
8. Serve hot.

Mutton ginger

Ingredients

Mutton leg 1 lb. small pieces
Onion 2 sliced
Ginger ½ cup finely chopped
Tomatoes 4 chopped
Green chili paste 1 table spoon
Coriander seeds powder ½ tea spoon
Cumin seeds powder ½ tea spoon
Turmeric powder ½ tea spoon
Five spice powder or garam masala powder ½ tea spoon
Salt to taste
Oil ½ cup

Directions

1. Fry onion in oil till golden brown.
2. Add tomatoes and green chili paste and fry.
3. Add mutton and fry.
4. Add rest of the ingredients except ginger and fry.
5. Add enough water for meat to get tender, mix well, simmer, cover and cook on low heat till meat gets tender.
6. Add finely chopped ginger and serve hot with rice.

Mutton BBQ kebab

Ingredients

Mutton leg 1 lb. small pieces
Yogurt ¼ cup
Lemon juice 3 table spoons
Paprika 1 table spoon
Cilantro 1 table spoon
Meat tenderizer 1 tea spoon
Ginger powder 1 table spoon
White pepper 1 tea spoon
Salt to taste

Directions

1. Marinade mutton in all the listed ingredients for 24 hours.
2. Thread mutton pieces over skewers and grill over charcoal till done.
3. Serve hot.

Mutton with peas

Ingredients

Mutton leg 1 lb. small pieces
Onion 1 sliced
Peas 1 cup
Tomatoes 4 chopped
Ginger and garlic paste 2 table spoons
Five spice powder or garam masala powder ½ tea spoon
Red chili powder 1 tea spoon
Cumin seeds powder 1 tea spoon
Coriander seeds powder 1 tea spoon
Turmeric powder ½ tea spoon
Salt to taste
Oil ½ cup

Directions

1. Fry onion in oil till golden brown.
2. Add tomatoes and cook till mushy.
3. Add rest of the ingredients except peas and fry.
4. Add enough water for meat to get tender and to have enough gravy.
5. Add peas and cook for five to ten more minutes.
6. Serve hot with rice.

Mutton with capsicum

Ingredients

Mutton leg 1 lb. small pieces
Capsicum 1 cup diced
Onion 1 sliced
Tomatoes 3 chopped
Ginger and garlic paste 2 table spoons
Herbs and spices of choice
Salt to taste
Oil ½ cup

Directions

1. Fry onion in oil till golden brown.
2. Add tomatoes and fry till mushy.
3. Add rest of the ingredients except capsicum and fry.
4. Add enough water needed to get mutton tender.
5. Add capsicum and cook for few more minutes.
6. Serve hot with rice.

Mutton and almond curry

Ingredients

Mutton leg 1 lb. small pieces
Onion 2 fried golden brown
Yogurt 1 cup
Almonds ½ cup blanched and roasted
Cilantro 1 table spoon
Green chili 1
Ginger l inch piece
Garlic Cloves 8
Salt and pepper to taste
Herbs and spices of choice 1 table spoon
Oil ½ cup

Directions

1. Blend fried onion with yogurt, ginger, garlic, cilantro and almonds.
2. Add these to a pan and fry.
3. Add mutton and fry.
4. Add rest of the ingredients and enough water for meat to get tender.
5. Mix well, cover, simmer and cook on low heat till mutton gets tender.
6. Serve hot with rice.

Conclusion

Thank you again for downloading this book!

I hope this book was able to help you to understand the gluten free world and how it can help you in your overall health

The next step is to the information and plans in your day to day food.

www.ingramcontent.com/pod-product-compliance
Lightning Source LLC
Chambersburg PA
CBHW071440070526
44578CB00001B/157